'This marvelous book by Ben Hine, PhD, is not for beginners. It is an elegant, scholarly text that goes far beyond describing the destructive relationships among family members who are experiencing parental alienation. Dr. Hine explores the social, psychological, legal, and political contexts that envelop every case of this unhappy mental condition. For example, he shows how other psychological concepts – attachment theory, psychoanalysis, family systems, and interpersonal acceptance-rejection theory – create a framework for understanding alienation. And he explores how the broad landscape – such as the ecosystem and macrosystem – plays out in different countries. And there is much more in this book that will enlighten family members, mental health and legal professionals, legislators, and policy-makers.'

William Bernet, *MD, Professor Emeritus, Department of Psychiatry and Behavioral Sciences, Vanderbilt University School of Medicine, Nashville, Tennessee, USA*

'Understanding Parental Alienation: Theoretical Insights, and Practical Solutions is a clear, balanced, and trustworthy examination of one of the most complex issues in family dynamics and family law. Accessible yet scientifically rigorous, it is an invaluable resource for seasoned practitioners and those just beginning to encounter parental alienation alike – a must-have resource that readers will find themselves returning to over and over again.'

Yvonne Parnell, *psychoanalyst, registered psychologist and Director of the Family Bridges Institute*

Ben Hine draws on personal experience and strong academic credentials to document parental alienation as a serious form of psychological abuse. In this detailed review of the scientific literature, Hine describes a nuanced and empirically grounded understanding of parental alienation as a relational outcome rather than a clinical diagnosis. Hine offers heartfelt descriptions of the impact on children, targeted parents, and extended family members, but he doesn't stop there. Speaking directly to victims as a survivor, Hine provides direct advice to children caught up in alienating parental battles. He then offers empirically based recommendations for mental health providers and the architects of public policy.

Demosthenes Lorandos, *PhD, JD, licensed psychologist, attorney at law*

Understanding Parental Alienation

Understanding Parental Alienation offers a clear, accessible starting point for anyone trying to make sense of parental alienation (PA): what it is, how it develops, and why it causes such profound harm. Opening with a grounded, user-friendly explanation of the phenomenon, the book demystifies PA without minimising its seriousness, setting the stage for a deeper exploration of its emotional, psychological, and legal dimensions.

From there, the book moves into a comprehensive examination of why parental alienation happens. Drawing on attachment theory to family-violence frameworks, it brings together leading theoretical insights to illuminate the mechanisms that drive bond-breaking between parents and children. This book expands beyond previous work to examine the wider ecosystem around PA, including the role of new partners, extended family members, complex sibling dynamics, and the systems that enable the abuse to take place.

The book then shifts to impact: analysing the short- and long-term consequences for every actor involved – children, targeted parents, alienating parents, siblings, and professionals encountering PA in practice. Finally, the book offers extensive practical guidance. It equips parents, practitioners, and policymakers with concrete, research-rooted strategies for recognising alienating behaviours and responding effectively. Alongside general principles for prevention and intervention, it includes tailored advice not only for affected parents but also for children and young people living through these dynamics.

Accessible, yet academically robust, *Understanding Parental Alienation* is a multi-purpose guide for mental health professionals, legal practitioners, family-court personnel, and families navigating post-separation conflict. It delivers the foundational knowledge and practical tools needed to understand this complex issue and to begin changing it.

Benjamin Hine, PhD, CPsychol, FHEA, is Professor of Applied Psychology at the University of West London and a leading expert in PA and domestic abuse. His extensive research on PA explores the psychological, societal, and legal dimensions of alienating behaviours, informed by both academic rigour and personal experience, having lived through parental alienation during his own childhood. Professor Hine's firsthand insight into the emotional and relational impacts of PA, paired with his academic experience, uniquely qualifies him to write this book.

Understanding Parental Alienation

Theoretical Insights and Practical Strategies

Benjamin Hine

Routledge
Taylor & Francis Group
LONDON AND NEW YORK

Designed cover image: Getty Images @Prostock-Studio

First published 2026
by Routledge
4 Park Square, Milton Park, Abingdon, Oxon OX14 4RN

and by Routledge
605 Third Avenue, New York, NY 10158

Routledge is an imprint of the Taylor & Francis Group, an informa business

British Library Cataloguing-in-Publication Data
A catalogue record for this book is available from the British Library

ISBN: 978-1-041-05005-6 (hbk)
ISBN: 978-1-041-05004-9 (pbk)
ISBN: 978-1-003-63094-4 (ebk)

DOI: 10.4324/9781003630944

Typeset in Optima
by Apex CoVantage, LLC

Contents

Acknowledgements

I want to thank my wife, Gemma. She has supported me at every step of my own PA journey; she is my rock, and I would not be alive today if it weren't for her.

To my children, thank you for anchoring me in love. Your presence is my daily reminder of all that is good, and your laughter and resilience have been the greatest motivation behind this work.

To my parents, for your courage in allowing your stories to be shared with honesty and vulnerability. You brought humanity into these pages and helped ensure that the theory never lost touch with the lived experience.

To my grandmother Pam, a steadfast source of support through every phase of life. Your calm wisdom and enduring presence have meant more than words can capture.

To my sister Sophie, for walking every step of this journey with me. Our shared history has been both a source of strength and solidarity. And to the rest of my brilliant, noisy, ever-supportive siblings, thank you for reminding me that families, no matter how complex, can still be full of laughter, chaos, and love.

To the organisations, professional bodies, and individuals, many of whom are referenced within this book, who have contributed your expertise and insights. Your input has been instrumental in shaping an evidence-based and compassionate understanding of this issue.

I would also like to thank Dr Jen Mayer and the University of West London for supporting this work when it is not always easy to do so.

And, to the hundreds of parents, children, grandparents, extended family members, and partners who have shared your stories with me over the last five years, this book owes its deepest truths to your voices. Your courage in telling the hardest stories and your unwavering push for justice have been both humbling and inspiring.

Preface – My Journey

My father describes the day I was born as one of the happiest days of his life – and it looks that way from the pictures I have seen. And for some time after my birth, my father, my mother, and I existed as a happy family of three, with close, loving parent–child relationships. However, within just a few years, my parents' relationship had deteriorated significantly for several reasons, including my mother's degenerative illness (multiple sclerosis) being hidden from all parties by my maternal grandparents.

One seemingly normal day, the actions of those grandparents brought an end to the relationship. Whilst my father was at work, they came and took my mother and me away from the home, along with all of the furniture, leaving a note for my father that he was no longer needed, except to pay child maintenance. Naturally, and following the intense shock and confusion that followed, my parents filed for divorce.

The four-year family court process that ensued left deep scars on all those involved, in large part due to the incredibly traumatising nature of a process that, whilst supposedly trying to "do the best for the child," became a fierce battleground between the two parties: my dad and step-mum on one side and my mother and maternal grandparents on the other – with me stuck in the middle. There is no doubt in my mind that all actions taken across that time were driven by love and a genuine desire to see me happy. Sadly, that did not always translate.

This was no more so the case than in how those grandparents, and to some extent my mother, went to great lengths to turn me against my father and to disrupt our relationship through a variety of means, including lies, verbal abuse, and coercive behaviours. I remember being made to feel deeply conflicted about showing loyalty or love towards him, my own father, or for forming new bonds with my stepmother. It placed deep psychological strain on me, as a child stuck between the two conflicting families.

That court case eventually ended when my grandparents and mother decided to withdraw the custody claim just two days before the final verdict was due, as a result of a cancer diagnosis for my grandmother that then rendered both my mother and grandparents unable to care for me. However, by that point, the damage had already been done.

They were left bitter and resentful, my father and stepmother were financially and emotionally broken, and I was left dazed and confused. The process had absolutely decimated my father, mainly due to the sustained attack on his role as a safe, loving parent.

His fight was rewarded, however. I moved into a new family home with him, my stepmother and my stepsister in 1998, and we began building new relationships. During subsequent years, my two half-siblings were born, and everybody continuously adjusted and adapted to life as a family of six.

But the scars from that process remained, and it greatly affected my ability to then support my mother, whom I also, of course, deeply loved, through her terminal illness, and then to deal with the subsequent grief after her passing when I was 18 years old. Indeed, it was due to the crippling "war" between the two families that meant that, when it became clear that my mother's journey was at an end, I was left to comfort her in the hospital alone. I then spent years grappling with severe mental health issues, many of which I have now been able to trace back to my parents' separation and everything that followed, including being alone in the hospital with my mother as she passed.

Those experiences have also greatly affected other relationships in my life, including my marriage, which has often been placed under significant strain due to my poor mental health and difficulty processing past trauma. This has been no more evident than in my current role as a father myself, as I have struggled to form relationships with my own children due to the experiences I had earlier in life.

Indeed, it is only in the last five years that I have begun to understand and truly process my experiences and, thankfully, to heal. Indeed, I owe a great deal to professionals who have not only helped me to unpick and dissect the behaviours I was subjected to, but to identify and tackle the relationships they have had with my present behaviour and psychopathy.

One of my main discoveries, both as an individual and an academic, was that what happened between my father and me had a name – *parental alienation*. It has subsequently become the driving force in my career to objectively, scientifically, and rationally explore and understand as much about this process as possible – and subsequently educate and inform evidence-based policy and practice in this area.

My father and I are still dealing with our wounds to this day, as is the case for many parents (including both mothers and fathers) and children who have been subject to a process where a child is "turned against" the other parent. Thankfully, I have a fantastic, loving relationship with my own children, and have had the chance to repair the relationship with my father, as he now occupies his grandfather (or more affectionately "popsie") role (and brilliantly too!).

However, many parents are not as "lucky" as my father and I; many remain alienated from their children to this day, and/or severely mentally ill, or dead from suicide. I also sadly never got to have these conversations with my mother due to her illness, or either of my maternal grandparents, who died when I was 8 and 13.

It is therefore my hope that this book provides not only a source of knowledge but also of support for all those affected by this complex and deeply damaging phenomenon. It is only through continually updating our understanding of these behaviours that we can begin to ensure that parents, children, and all those affected are protected from serious and long-lasting harm.

INTRODUCTION

Families are, at their best, environments of safety, love, and continuity; spaces where children develop enduring bonds with both parents and a broader network of caregivers. Yet, in some cases, these vital relationships become disrupted, not by natural drift or mutual conflict, but through a systematic process that distorts a child's perception of one parent and undermines the parent–child bond. This phenomenon, widely recognised as parental alienation (PA), reflects a pattern of behaviours and relational dynamics that can result in the unjustified rejection of one parent by a child, most commonly following separation or divorce. The consequences are often profound, long-lasting, and emotionally devastating.

Understanding Parental Alienation: Theoretical Insights and Practical Strategies seeks to provide a comprehensive and interdisciplinary account of this complex and often misunderstood issue. Going beyond surface-level interpretations, this book situates parental alienation within broader frameworks of psychological manipulation, family violence, attachment disruption, and relational trauma. It examines how parental alienation is enacted, its effects on children, parents, and extended families, and how it is recognised, assessed, and contested within clinical and legal domains.

Across its chapters, this volume integrates theoretical exploration with practical application. Readers will find critical engagement with contested definitions, emerging debates in the academic literature, and real-world

DOI: 10.4324/9781003630944-1

strategies for addressing the emotional and legal challenges posed by parental alienation. The text provides insight into the lived experiences of alienated families, the evidentiary base supporting intervention, and the institutional barriers that continue to complicate identification and redress.

Ultimately, this book aims to equip parents, practitioners, legal professionals, and policymakers with both the conceptual tools and practical guidance necessary to respond effectively and compassionately to parental alienation. In doing so, it aspires to contribute to healthier familial outcomes, greater justice in family law, and a more robust public understanding of an issue that touches the lives of far too many.

OBJECTIVES OF THIS BOOK

This book aims to provide a definitive, evidence-based account of PA, addressing both its theoretical complexity and real-world impact. It brings together empirical research, clinical insight, and legal analysis to clarify what PA is, how it emerges, why it persists, and how it may be prevented or resolved. By drawing on multiple disciplinary perspectives – psychological, sociological, legal, and systemic – it offers a rigorous yet accessible framework for understanding and addressing this multifaceted issue.

The structure of the book reflects five overarching objectives:

1. *To establish a clear and contemporary understanding of parental alienation,* including its definition, measurable features, and distinction from other resist-refuse dynamics such as justified estrangement or enmeshment. Chapters 1–5 address these foundational questions by defining key terms, reviewing the scientific status of PA, exploring adjacent phenomena, and discussing both measurement and prevalence.
2. *To explore the motivations, dynamics, and theoretical underpinnings of PA,* including the behaviours of alienating parents, the child's role, and the wider cultural, familial, and relational contexts that sustain alienation. Chapters 6–9 examine the psychological and systemic factors that contribute to PA and explicitly position it within frameworks of coercive control and family violence.
3. *To map the impact of PA across different members of the family system,* including children, targeted parents, siblings, grandparents, and new partners. Chapters 10–12 analyse short- and long-term outcomes, with particular attention to psychological distress, identity disruption, and relational trauma.
4. *To provide a critical examination of institutional responses to PA,* particularly within legal systems. Chapters 13–19 focus on early intervention, family court engagement, legal processes, and therapeutic approaches, assessing both best practice and current limitations.
5. *To offer practical, evidence-informed guidance for those affected by PA,* including alienated parents, other family members, children, and

professionals. Chapters 20–22 deliver specific advice tailored to each stakeholder group, covering emotional wellbeing, legal navigation, relationship repair, and community roles.

The final chapter (Chapter 23) concludes by calling for systemic reform, increased public and professional awareness, and a more coherent, trauma-informed response to PA as a form of post-separation abuse.

By integrating research, theory, and applied knowledge, this book serves as a comprehensive resource for parents, legal and mental health professionals, policymakers, and scholars. Its goal is not only to inform but also to support and empower those navigating the complex realities of PA and to promote healthier outcomes for children and families worldwide.

HOW TO USE THIS BOOK

This book has been carefully written to remain accessible and supportive, without sacrificing intellectual rigour. As such, while it draws extensively on a broad base of empirical research, professional literature, and lived experience, the chapters are deliberately free from in-text academic referencing. Instead, each chapter presents a blended overview of the current evidence alongside the author's professional insights and practical guidance. This approach ensures that the material remains readable and engaging for a diverse audience, while still being grounded in contemporary scholarship and best practice.

Readers who wish to explore the research base in more depth are directed to the reference lists at the end of each chapter, as well as *Appendix A*, which lists a wide range of additional books in this space. For those seeking support services or signposting, *Appendix B* provides a curated list of organisations, websites, and agencies offering help across different jurisdictions.

The book is designed to be used flexibly. While it is structured thematically and sequentially, it does not need to be read cover-to-cover. Readers are encouraged to begin with the sections that most closely align with their current needs. For instance, those newly encountering parental alienation may benefit from early chapters that define the phenomenon and explore its emergence. Others, already entrenched in family court proceedings or emotional distress, may find greater value in the sections on legal strategy, mental health, or reunification.

Most chapters will resonate internationally, and the conceptual discussions, psychological insights, and practical strategies apply across borders. Where appropriate, references to international practice or global research perspectives are integrated.

In recognition of the emotional toll that PA can take, this book also includes dedicated chapters including advice on *self-care, emotional resilience*, and *support for children*. These sections are written with compassion and care, and aim to provide reassurance, validation, and tangible steps towards wellbeing.

Ultimately, this book is intended to serve as a practical, evidence-informed companion for navigating the challenges of parental alienation. Whether you are a parent, child, practitioner, legal professional, or concerned ally, the aim is to equip you with insight, understanding, and strategies that can support healing, restore connections, and promote justice.

A NOTE BEFORE WE BEGIN

Parental alienation is a subject that continues to attract both attention and controversy. While some question its validity or misuse in certain legal contexts, others argue that insufficient recognition of its dynamics has left children and families vulnerable to long-term harm. These debates, while important, have at times generated more heat than light, creating confusion, polarisation, and in some cases, inaction.

This book does not seek to silence debate but rather to ground it. It offers a measured, evidence-informed exploration of parental alienation, shaped by current research, professional experience, and the lived realities of those affected. It neither overstates the problem nor dismisses legitimate critiques. Instead, it aims to cut through the noise by acknowledging complexity, attending to nuance, and focusing continuously on the well-being of children and families.

Readers are encouraged to approach this text with openness and critical curiosity. You may find concepts here that challenge assumptions or reframe familiar issues. You may encounter perspectives that feel uncomfortable, or conversely, affirming. That is part of the process of engaging with an issue that, while still developing as a field of study, carries real and immediate consequences for the lives of many.

Whatever your role, whether you are a parent, practitioner, legal professional, student, or policymaker, this book is written for you. It is for those who want to understand parental alienation more deeply, to support those affected more effectively, and to contribute to a more just and compassionate response.

So with that, let us begin.

PART 1

WHAT IS PARENTAL ALIENATION?

1

DEFINING PARENTAL ALIENATION (PA) AND PARENTAL ALIENATING BEHAVIOURS (PABS)

Parental Alienation (PA) has long been subjected to an unfortunate and persistent myth: that it is conceptually vague, poorly defined, or even an unsubstantiated label with no place in serious academic, clinical, or legal discourse. Critics have at times argued that PA lacks a clear scientific foundation or that it is too contested to be reliably identified. These narratives, often fuelled by ideological resistance, outdated critiques, or confusion with earlier formulations such as Parental Alienation Syndrome (PAS), have contributed to harmful misunderstanding and minimisation of a very real form of psychological and relational abuse. This chapter aims to decisively dispel the notion that PA is inherently nebulous. Drawing upon a substantial and growing body of empirical research, this chapter presents a clear, operationalised definition of PA that distinguishes it from other types of parent–child contact problems, such as justified estrangement or loyalty conflicts (which will be discussed later in Chapter 3). It also introduces key conceptual distinctions, such as that between Parental Alienation and Parental Alienating Behaviours (PABs), to provide a comprehensive framework for understanding what PA is, how it occurs, and why it matters. In doing so, this chapter aims to establish definitive clarity in definitions.

DOI: 10.4324/9781003630944-3

PARENTAL ALIENATION (PA) AND PARENTAL ALIENATING BEHAVIOURS (PABS)

PA is increasingly recognised as a coherent and scientifically valid construct, though confusion has persisted due to its contested history and variable terminology. One of the most important clarifications in recent literature is the distinction between PA as an *outcome* and Parental Alienating Behaviours (PABs) as the *process* by which that outcome is produced. This distinction is fundamental to understanding, assessing, and responding appropriately to alienation dynamics in separated families.

Parental Alienation (PA): A Relational Outcome

At its core, parental alienation is a relational outcome in which a child, without legitimate justification, rejects or resists a relationship with one parent, commonly referred to as the targeted or alienated parent. This typically occurs in the context of a high-conflict separation or divorce and reflects the child's alignment with the other parent, often described as the alienating or aligned parent. Crucially, this rejection cannot be attributed to the targeted parent's behaviour (e.g., abuse, neglect, or demonstrable parenting deficits), but is instead driven by a sustained pattern of influence exerted by the alienating parent.

This phenomenon has been most clearly articulated by Bernet et al. (2022) who define PA as:

> One type of contact refusal, when a child – typically whose parents are engaged in a high-conflict separation or divorce – allies strongly with one parent and resists and rejects contact and/or a relationship with the other parent without legitimate justification. PA refers to the actions and attitudes manifested by the child. PA is brought on by the alienating behaviours of the parent with whom the child is aligned.

The key elements of this definition – contact refusal, lack of legitimate justification, and influence by alienating behaviours – are now widely regarded as the central tenets of PA. Indeed, although alternative definitions may exist, these core principles remain consistent across the literature. For example, some definitions take a broader stance, focusing less on pathology and more on behavioural influence and relational outcomes, and describe PA as "a situation whereby one parent has a negative influence on a child's relationship with the other parent and makes a deliberate effort to intervene and prevent the relationship from developing, continuing, or improving" (McCarten, 2022, p. 2).

Despite these variations in wording and emphasis, there is remarkable consistency in the underlying conceptualisation: PA is a patterned breakdown of a previously healthy parent–child relationship, occurring in the absence of abuse or neglect, and attributable to the manipulation of the child's perceptions by the other parent.

Parental Alienating Behaviours (PABs): The Causal Mechanism

Whereas PA refers to the observable outcome (i.e., the child's unjustified rejection), Parental Alienating Behaviours (PABs) describe the specific actions undertaken by the alienating parent, or, in some cases, other actors, such as extended family members, legal representatives, or professionals, that contribute to that rejection. As Rowlands (2019) succinctly puts it, PABs are "activities that contribute to the child's rejection of the alienated parent" (p. 317). These behaviours range from overt denigration and obstruction of contact to more covert forms of manipulation, such as instilling fear or guilt, creating false narratives, and fostering emotional enmeshment.

Empirical and clinical research has repeatedly shown that alienating parents engage in a consistent pattern of behaviours designed to erode the child's relationship with the other parent. These parental alienating behaviours (PABs) are now well documented. They are not isolated incidents but rather sustained and strategic actions that distort the child's perceptions and interfere with a healthy attachment to the targeted parent. The most commonly observed behaviours include:

1. *Bad-mouthing the rejected parent,* including making derogatory comments or blaming them for the family breakdown.
2. *Limiting the child's contact* with the rejected parent, either directly or by creating obstacles to visitation or communication.
3. *Interfering with the child's communications* with the rejected parent, such as blocking calls, reading messages, or refusing to pass on information.
4. *Limiting mention of the rejected parent,* including removing photographs or prohibiting discussion.
5. *Withholding approval when the child shows an interest* in the rejected parent, subtly discouraging affection or curiosity.
6. *Telling the child that the rejected parent does not love them,* thereby undermining the child's sense of safety and emotional security.
7. *Allowing or encouraging the child to choose between parents,* which places the burden of allegiance on the child and reinforces rejection.
8. *Creating the impression that the rejected parent is dangerous,* incompetent, or emotionally unstable.
9. *Forcing or pressuring the child to reject* the targeted parent, including through coercion, guilt, or emotional manipulation.
10. *Confiding in the child about adult topics,* such as legal matters or personal grievances, to gain their alliance.
11. *Asking the child to spy on the rejected parent,* blurring boundaries and encouraging betrayal.

12. *Asking the child to keep secrets* from the rejected parent, thereby damaging trust and transparency.
13. *Referring to the rejected parent by their first name*, diminishing their parental status and authority.
14. *Referring to a stepparent as "Mum" or "Dad,"* replacing the alienated parent's role in the child's life.
15. *Withholding medical, social, or academic information* from the rejected parent, excluding them from key areas of decision-making.
16. *Changing the child's name* to remove association with the rejected parent.
17. *Undermining the authority* of the rejected parent, including dismissing rules, decisions, or parental boundaries.

While the 17 behaviours listed above represent the most empirically established and commonly observed indicators of parental alienation, they are by no means exhaustive. Other behaviours, such as emotional blackmail, excessive gatekeeping, triangulation, micro-invalidations, or the strategic use of professional reports to discredit the targeted parent, have also been identified in clinical and research contexts. However, whether a particular behaviour constitutes alienation depends not solely on its occurrence but on its pattern, persistence, and context. For example, some actions may appear benign, or even protective, in isolation, but, when embedded in a sustained campaign to undermine the parent–child relationship, they take on a more sinister function. This nuanced issue of context, and the importance of distinguishing between justified and unjustified rejection, is discussed in detail in subsequent chapters.

Why the Distinction Matters

Understanding the difference between PA and PABs is not merely a matter of semantics; it has profound implications for clinical assessment, legal adjudication, and intervention planning. PA cannot be reliably inferred from contact refusal alone; it must be evaluated in the context of the broader behavioural pattern of the aligned parent, and the absence of legitimate reasons for rejection. Likewise, the presence of PABs does not automatically indicate that alienation has occurred, but it does suggest that the parent–child relationship is at risk of disruption and warrants professional scrutiny.

Moreover, this distinction facilitates clarity in communication across disciplines. Mental health professionals, legal practitioners, and child protection workers often approach these cases from different vantage points; anchoring definitions in the distinction between behaviour and outcome enhances multidisciplinary coherence and safeguards against misinterpretation.

LEVELS OF PARENTAL ALIENATION: MILD, MODERATE, AND SEVERE

Parental alienation is not a binary phenomenon. Rather than being either present or absent, it is more accurately conceptualised along a spectrum of severity, ranging from mild to moderate to severe, depending on the intensity, persistence, and relational impact of the alienating dynamics. This graduated understanding is critical for both accurate assessment and the tailoring of appropriate interventions. As McCarten and others have argued, the severity of alienation is not merely descriptive; it is diagnostic in determining the urgency and type of response required.

Importantly, describing a case as involving "mild" parental alienation does not imply that the harm is insignificant. Much like the staging of a progressive illness, early-stage alienation may be less entrenched but remains clinically serious, particularly if it continues unaddressed. The spectrum helps professionals gauge where the child is in the alienation process, how accessible the child's attachment system is to repair, and what level of professional intervention may be warranted.

Mild Parental Alienation

At the mild stage, children may exhibit early signs of alienation, such as withdrawal, anxiety during transitions, or subtle alignment with the alienating parent. They may still express love or affection for the alienated parent in private, but show reluctance to do so openly, particularly when under the influence or surveillance of the alienating parent. Resistance to visitation may occur, especially during transitions, but, once contact is re-established, the child typically re-engages positively and enjoys time with the alienated parent. The alienating behaviours are often intermittent, less overt, or minimised, and the child's internal conflict remains visible. This level is often responsive to low-intensity interventions, such as therapeutic mediation, psychoeducation, or parent–child counselling.

Moderate Parental Alienation

In moderate cases, the alienating dynamic has become more consolidated, and the child begins to adopt more entrenched negative views of the alienated parent. Contact resistance intensifies, transitions become more fraught, and the child may display overt hostility, defiance, or rejection behaviours. Although the child may still participate in activities with the alienated parent, these are accompanied by a reluctant or conflicted emotional tone, and any enjoyment is often cognitively or emotionally disavowed. Positive memories may be dismissed, and the child begins to echo unfounded or exaggerated criticisms that are often traceable to the alienating parent's narrative.

This stage often requires structured therapeutic intervention, sometimes including court-mandated reunification efforts or coordinated mental health involvement across both households.

Severe Parental Alienation

Severe parental alienation is characterised by a complete rupture of the parent–child relationship. The child may refuse all contact, present a black-and-white view of the alienated parent, and exhibit profound emotional detachment or hostility, sometimes bordering on cruelty, without visible guilt or ambivalence. Affection, warmth, or past relational memories are denied or rewritten, and the child may insist they have independently formed these views, despite obvious inconsistencies or developmental implausibilities. At this level, alienating behaviours are typically frequent, overt, and institutionalised, involving legal strategies, professional enmeshment, or systemic collusion. Intervention becomes significantly more complex and may necessitate intensive, court-directed therapeutic responses, sometimes including temporary custodial transfer or structured reintegration protocols.

THE HISTORY OF PA AND CURRENT THINKING

Understanding where the concept of Parental Alienation (PA) has come from is vital for grasping both its current status and the nature of the controversies that continue to surround it. The evolution of PA theory reflects broader shifts in psychological, legal, and sociopolitical thinking, particularly regarding how family conflict, coercion, and post-separation abuse are understood and addressed.

Origins: Parental Alienation Syndrome (PAS)

The modern conceptualisation of PA has its roots in the work of American child psychiatrist Richard A. Gardner, who, in the 1980s, introduced the controversial notion of *Parental Alienation Syndrome* (PAS). Gardner described PAS as a psychological disorder in which a child – typically one involved in a conflictual custody dispute – unjustifiably rejects one parent as a result of the psychological manipulation of the other. While Gardner's introduction of PAS brought significant attention to the phenomenon of unjustified parent–child rejection, his work has since attracted considerable criticism on several fronts.

First, PAS lacked empirical rigour. It was based largely on Gardner's clinical impressions and anecdotal observations, rather than on systematic, peer-reviewed research. This absence of a solid evidence base led many scholars to question its validity as a distinct psychiatric diagnosis. Critics argued that existing frameworks – such as attachment theory or family systems theory – offered more robust ways to conceptualise the phenomenon without pathologising children or parents.

Second, PAS has been widely criticised for perpetuating gender stereotypes. Gardner often characterised mothers as the primary alienators and fathers as the typical victims. This gendered framing has been robustly challenged by subsequent empirical research showing that alienating behaviours can be perpetrated by *any* parent or caregiver, regardless of gender or custody status.

Third, PAS became deeply problematic in legal contexts. It was sometimes invoked in ways that silenced legitimate claims of abuse or domestic violence. In some custody disputes, abusive parents used PAS as a legal strategy to discredit the other parent's concerns and secure custody, despite clear evidence of harm. This led to widespread concern that PAS could be weaponised to the detriment of both children and protective parents.

Fourth, the context of PAS's development raises important ethical questions. Gardner formulated the syndrome during a time of major cultural shifts in divorce, custody, and child protection – particularly as allegations of abuse, including sexual abuse, were increasing in family courts. Gardner argued that many such allegations were false and implanted by vindictive parents, usually mothers. While this may have reflected some cases, critics argue that this framing risked invalidating genuine disclosures of abuse and disproportionately cast suspicion on maternal caregivers.

Finally, Gardner's broader body of work has been subject to serious ethical scrutiny. His writings on paedophilia and child–adult sexual relationships were widely regarded as inappropriate and, in some cases, deeply disturbing (Dallam, 1999). This has further tainted the credibility of PAS in professional and academic circles.

Moving Forward: The Shift to PA and PABs

In light of these controversies, the field has gradually shifted away from the idea of *Parental Alienation Syndrome* and towards a more nuanced and empirically grounded understanding of *Parental Alienation* as a relational *outcome* rather than a clinical diagnosis. Contemporary researchers and practitioners now conceptualise PA as the unjustified rejection of a parent, brought about by a pattern of alienating behaviours, commonly referred to as *Parental Alienating Behaviours* (PABs).

This reframing has been driven by two key insights:

- First, that PA is not a syndrome but a form of psychological and relational abuse that emerges in the context of high-conflict family dynamics, particularly post-separation.
- Second, that PABs are the mechanisms by which the alienation is enacted. These behaviours can include denigration, emotional

manipulation, restriction of contact, or even false allegations, and they must be understood within their broader context.

The move away from a diagnostic model is also reflected in the clinical literature. Rather than seeking to include PAS as a standalone disorder in diagnostic manuals, many professionals now support recognising PA-related dynamics under broader relational categories. For example, *"Parental Alienation Relational Problem"* has been proposed for inclusion in the DSM-5-TR's section on *Other Conditions That May Be a Focus of Clinical Attention*. This shift allows for clinical recognition and intervention without pathologising the child or relying on a controversial diagnostic label.

It is important to note, however, that this movement away from PAS does *not* represent a rejection of the core phenomenon. Rather, it reflects a more accurate and scientifically robust understanding; one that recognises PA as a pattern of behaviour and a relational problem, not a fixed or inherent psychiatric disorder. This change in framing not only aligns with contemporary models of family violence and coercive control but also facilitates more responsible use of PA concepts in legal, therapeutic, and policy contexts.

CURRENT CONSENSUS

Despite continued ideological resistance in some quarters, the current consensus among leading researchers is clear: Parental Alienation is a real and highly damaging phenomenon. It is best understood through empirical evidence, behavioural patterns, and relational outcomes, rather than through outdated clinical diagnoses. The modern focus is on identifying, assessing, and interrupting the alienating process, whether or not the child has developed a fully entrenched rejection of the targeted parent. This includes examining the behaviours involved, the motivations driving them, and the systemic responses (or failures) that allow them to persist.

The evolution from PAS to PA and PABs represents progress: a shift from controversial origins to a maturing scientific field increasingly capable of addressing the complex and nuanced realities of family breakdown and post-separation abuse.

BIBLIOGRAPHY

Bernet, W., Baker, A. J., & Adkins, K. L. (2022). Definitions and terminology regarding child alignments, estrangement, and alienation: A survey of custody evaluators. *Journal of Forensic Sciences*, *67*(1), 279–288. https://doi.org/10.1111/1556-4029.14868

Bernet, W., Wamboldt, M. Z., & Narrow, W. E. (2016). Child affected by parental relationship distress. *Child and Adolescent Psychiatry*, *55*, 571–579. https://doi.org/10.1016/j.jaac.2016.04.018

Dallam, S. J. (1999). Parental alienation syndrome: Is it scientific? In E. S. Charles & L. Crook (Eds.), *Expose: The failure of family courts to protect children from abuse in custody disputes*. Los Gatos, CA: Our Children Our Children Charitable Foundation.

Haines, J., Matthewson, M., & Turnbull, M. (2019). *Understanding and managing parental alienation: A guide to assessment and intervention*. Routledge.

Harman, J. J., Bernet, W., & Harman, J. (2019). Parental alienation: The blossoming of a field of study. *Current Directions in Psychological Science*, *28*(2), 212–217. https://doi.org/10.1177/0963721419827271

Harman, J. J., & Matthewson, M. (2020). Parental alienation: How is it done. In D. Lorandos & W. Bernet (Eds.), *Parental alienation – science and law*. Charles C Thomas Publisher, Ltd.

Harman, J. J., Warshak, R., Lorandos, D., & Florian, M. J. (2022). Developmental psychology and the scientific status of parental alienation. *Developmental Psychology*. https://doi.org/10.1037/dev0001404

Hine, B. A. (2024). Parental alienation – What do we know, and what do we (urgently) need to know? A narrative review. *Partner Abuse*, 15(3), 362–396. https://doi.org/10.1891/PA-2023-0015

Marques, T. M., Narciso, I., & Ferreira, L. C. (2020). Empirical research on parental alienation: A descriptive literature review. *Children and Youth Services Review*, *119*, 1–12. https://doi.org/10.1016/j.childyouth.2020.105572

McCarten, D. (2022). *Parental alienation: An evidence-based approach*. Routledge.

Meier, J. S. (2009). A historical perspective on parental alienation syndrome and parental alienation. *Journal of Child Custody*, *6*, 232–257. https://doi.org/10.1080/15379410903084681

Rowlands, G. A. (2019). Parental alienation: A measurement tool. *Divorce & Remarriage*, *60*, 316–331. https://doi.org/10.1080/10502556.2018.1546031

2

THE SCIENTIFIC STATUS OF PA

As established in Chapter 1, the movement away from Parental Alienation Syndrome (PAS) towards the more robust and operationalised concept of Parental Alienation (PA) reflects not only theoretical refinement but also a broader shift towards scientific credibility. Over the past decade, in particular, the field has undergone a notable transformation, marked by a growing number of peer-reviewed studies, validated assessment tools, and interdisciplinary analyses. Scholars such as Jennifer Harman have argued that the literature has now reached a "critical mass" in terms of methodological quality and empirical consistency, firmly establishing PA as a legitimate phenomenon of study. This chapter thus briefly outlines the current scientific status of PA, summarising the central claims made by critics, and evaluating them against this increasingly well-developed evidence base. While later chapters in this book will explore the application of specific models, measurements, and interventions in greater depth, our purpose here is more limited: to demonstrate that PA meets the criteria of a scientifically valid construct, and that continued denial of its reality is no longer tenable.

KEY CRITICISMS OF THE SCIENTIFIC STATUS OF PARENTAL ALIENATION

Despite the field's ongoing movement away from Parental Alienation Syndrome (PAS) and towards a more refined and empirically grounded

DOI: 10.4324/9781003630944-4

concept of Parental Alienation (PA), significant debate remains about its scientific legitimacy. Critics from various academic, legal, and clinical backgrounds have raised a number of recurring concerns, which can broadly be summarised under the following themes:

1. **Lack of Rigorous Empirical Evidence**
   One of the most frequently cited critiques is that the empirical foundation of PA is insufficient. Scholars such as Madelyn Milchman, Jean Mercer, John Myers, and Joan Meier argue that much of the literature relies heavily on anecdotal case studies, retrospective accounts, or clinical impressions, rather than systematic, peer-reviewed research. They contend that, without a clearly operationalised and consistently applied definition, the phenomenon cannot be meaningfully measured or validated at scale.
2. **Overapplication and Misuse of the Concept**
   A second major concern relates to the perceived overextension of the PA label. Critics argue that PA is sometimes applied indiscriminately to any instance in which a child resists or refuses contact with a parent, without adequate differential assessment. This overapplication risks conflating PA with other forms of contact resistance, such as justified estrangement, loyalty conflicts, or protective gatekeeping in the context of abuse. The fear is that such conflation diminishes the concept's diagnostic clarity and allows it to be misused in both clinical and legal settings.
3. **Bias in Early Foundations and Contemporary Research**
   Sceptics also point to ideological or professional biases that may have influenced the early development and ongoing promotion of PA. Particular attention is often given to Richard Gardner's legacy and his personal investment in defining PAS as a psychiatric disorder. Even though modern research has largely moved beyond Gardner's original framing, critics suggest that the field remains shaped by partisan narratives, particularly in adversarial legal contexts, and caution against confirmation bias in research and expert testimony.

Overcoming Misinformation: The Empirical Foundation of PA

Despite the controversies outlined above, it is now clear that a significant portion of the criticism aimed at parental alienation (PA) stems not from genuine scholarly disagreement but from persistent misinformation, flawed methodology, or ideologically driven narratives. As Harman et al. (2022) powerfully argue, the continued dismissal of PA as unscientific is not only outdated but also harmful. Their comprehensive systematic review identified 213 empirical studies on PA, published in ten languages and using diverse methodologies, including qualitative, quantitative, and mixed-methods approaches. Importantly, nearly 40% of these studies were published since 2016, signalling a rapid acceleration in the maturity and rigour of the field.

Critics often rely on outdated or narrow reviews such as Saini et al. (2016), which applied a medical evaluation tool (GRADE) ill-suited to the diversity of research in developmental and psychological sciences. Harman et al. demonstrate that such critiques often overlook the complexity of the field and ignore a broad body of research that supports PA as a legitimate and empirically grounded construct. They conclude unequivocally:

> Given that nearly 40% of the studies on PA have been published since 2016, it falls to scholars and practitioners to update their knowledge about PA and incorporate these scientific advances. It is no longer tenable to dismiss the field as lacking in scientific status. Only by recognizing the legitimacy of PA scholarship will developmental psychology sustain and enhance understanding of how and why parent–child relationships break down in the wake of interparental conflict, separation, and divorce.
>
> (Harman et al., 2022, p. 1908)

This view is echoed and extended in the doctoral work of Joshua Marsden, who further dismantles the claim that PA lacks scientific grounding. Marsden provides a detailed assessment of the literature, addresses definitional clarity, critiques commonly misunderstood aspects of the concept, and strongly defends the empirical status of PA against its detractors. Like Harman, Marsden highlights that many of the criticisms rest on misinterpretations of what PA is, and is not, and fail to engage with the field's robust empirical foundations.

Together, Harman et al. and Marsden represent a decisive shift in the discourse, moving from defensiveness to affirmation. This chapter has not attempted to catalogue all the existing studies or models; that is the work of the chapters that follow. Instead, it has established the core truth that should now be indisputable: Parental Alienation is a scientifically validated concept, built on a growing and diverse evidence base, and deserving of recognition as a legitimate subject of academic inquiry and professional intervention.

BIBLIOGRAPHY

Aichenbaum, Y., Bernet, W., Brzosowski, B., Cedervall, B., Hellstern, B., Korosi, S., Ludmer, B., Marcus, P., & Mendoza-Amaro, A. (2023). *An analysis of the report of the special rapporteur on violence against women and girls, its causes and consequences.* https://static1.squarespace.com/static/652b4267cc223c56e83ab445/t/654056fdbe05f47265e9f667/1698715390344/Analysis-Report-Special-Rapporteur-2023-06-02.pdf

Aichenbaum, Y., Bernet, W., Cedervall, B., Harman, J. J., Mendoza-Amaro, A., & Sheery, A. (2023). *A comprehensive review of misinformation and other inaccuracies in challegning parental alienation: New directions for professional and parents.* https://static1.squarespace.com/static/652b4267cc223c56e83ab445/t/65458eb7e8169324d7df6734/1699057338096/Analysis-of-Mercer-Drew-2023-04-04.pdf

Bernet, W. (2020). Parental alienation and misinformation proliferation. *Family Court Review, 58*, 293–307. https://doi.org/10.1111/fcre.12473

Bernet, W. (2023). Recurrent misinformation regarding parental alienation theory. *The American Journal of Family Therapy*, *51*, 334–355. https://doi.org/10.1080/01926187.2021.1972494

Bernet, W., & Xu, S. (2023). Scholarly rumors: Citation analysis of vast misinformation regarding parental alienation theory. *Behavioral Sciences and the Law*, *45*, 231–245. https://doi.org/10.1002/bsl.2605

Harman, J. J., Warshak, R., Lorandos, D., & Florian, M. J. (2022). Developmental psychology and the scientific status of parental alienation. *Developmental Psychology*, *58*(10), 1887–1911. https://doi.org/10.1037/dev0001404

Hine, B. A. (2024). Parental alienation – What do we know, and what do we (urgently) need to know? A narrative review. *Partner Abuse*, *15*(3), 362–396. https://doi.org/10.1891/PA-2023-0015

Marsden, J. (2024). *The scientific rigour of parental alienation studies: A quality assessment of the peer-reviewed research*. Colorado: Colorado State University.

Meier, J. S. (2022). Questioning the scientific validity of parental aleination in abuse cases. In J. Mercer & M. Drew (Eds.), *Challenging parental alienation: New directions for practitioners and parents* (pp. 216–235). Routledge.

Mercer, J. (2021). Critiquing assumptions about parental alienation: Part 1. The analogy with family violence. *Journal of Family Trauma, Child Custody & Child Development*, 1–17. https://doi.org/10.1080/26904586.2021.1957057

Mercer, J. (2022a). Critiquing assumptions about parental alienation: Part 2. Causes of psychological harms. *Journal of Family Trauma, Child Custody & Child Development*, 1–18. https://doi.org/10.1080/26904586.2021.1957058

Mercer, J. (2022b). Parental alienation, science, and pseudoscience. In J. Mercer & M. Drew (Eds.), *Challenging parental alienation: New directions for professionals and parents* (pp. 236–248). Routledge.

Mercer, J., & Drew, M. (2022). *Challenging parental alienation: New directions for professionals and parents*. Routledge.

Milchman, M. S. (2019). How far has parental alienation research progressed toward achieving scientific validity? *Journal of Child Custody*, *16*, 115–139. https://doi.org/10.1080/15379418.2019.1614511

Milchman, M. S., Geffner, R., & Meier, J. S. (2020a). Ideology and rhetoric replace science and reason in some parental alienation literature and advocacy: A critique. *Family Court Review*, *58*, 340–361. https://doi.org/10.1111/fcre.12476

Milchman, M. S., Geffner, R., & Meier, J. S. (2020b). Putting science and reasoning back into the "parental alienation" discussion: Reply to Bernet, Robb, Lorandos, and Garber. *Family Court Review*, *58*, 375–385. https://doi.org/10.1111/fcre.12477

Saini, M., Johnston, J. R., Fidler, B. J., & Bala, N. (2016). *Empirical studies of alienation* (Vol. 2, pp. 374–430). New York, NY: Oxford University Press.

3

UNDERSTANDING OTHER RESIST–REFUSE DYNAMICS

One of the most persistent criticisms of parental alienation (PA) theory is that it is allegedly over-applied, used indiscriminately to explain any instance in which a child resists or refuses contact with a parent. As outlined in Chapter 1, however, PA is a specific relational outcome arising from sustained alienating behaviours in the absence of legitimate reasons for rejection. When properly understood, PA is not a catch-all label but a phenomenon that must always be assessed in context. That context, psychological, relational, and situational, is essential to determining whether a child's rejection stems from alienation or from other dynamics. While Chapter 5 will explore how this complexity is addressed through structured measurement and assessment tools, the current chapter focuses on an equally important task: exploring the range of alternative explanations for contact refusal. These include, but are not limited to, justified estrangement, loyalty conflicts, enmeshment, and developmental responses to high-conflict separation. By clearly delineating these dynamics, this chapter aims to sharpen the conceptual boundaries of PA and directly address the claim that it is applied too broadly. In doing so, it reinforces the necessity of careful, evidence-informed differentiation in both clinical and legal contexts.

DOI: 10.4324/9781003630944-5

CONTEXT IS CRITICAL

As detailed in Chapter 1, PA is a specific form of psychological and relational abuse that involves the unjustified rejection of a parent, typically following separation or divorce, driven by the sustained behaviours of an alienating parent. However, this specificity is frequently misunderstood or misrepresented. One of the most persistent critiques of PA theory is that it is over-applied, such that any form of contact resistance is reflexively attributed to alienation. This is a mischaracterisation that this chapter aims to confront directly.

Children's resistance to contact with a parent is a behaviour that *requires* explanation. Evolutionary psychology and attachment theory both suggest that children are biologically and psychologically predisposed to form and maintain attachments to caregivers, even in contexts of significant dysfunction. Thus, when a child resists or refuses contact with a parent, this is atypical and signals that something meaningful is occurring in the family system. The key task for professionals is to determine *what* that something is. PA is one possibility, *but it is not the only one*. Understanding PA correctly means understanding what it is *not*, and recognising the full range of other dynamics that can lead to contact problems is essential to that process.

Typical and Developmentally Expected Resistance

It is important to first acknowledge that not all resistance or preference is pathological. In intact families, or following separation, children may express preferences for one parent over another or may occasionally resist contact altogether. These dynamics can arise from a variety of developmentally normal factors, including:

- Separation anxiety, particularly among younger children
- Adolescent individuation, during which teenagers seek autonomy and may push back against parental authority
- Personality mismatches, where a child simply gets along better with one parent
- Parenting style differences, such as preferring a more lenient or playful parent
- Short-term disruptions or stressors, such as moving homes or transitions between households

These forms of resistance are usually mild, transient, and do not involve the deep-seated hostility, fear, or moral denigration of the targeted parent that characterises PA. In most cases, they resolve naturally or with light-touch support and do not indicate a need for formal intervention.

Justified Estrangement

In contrast to PA, justified estrangement occurs when a child refuses contact with a parent due to legitimate concerns, such as abuse, neglect, or severely deficient parenting. In these cases, the child's rejection is proportionate to actual experiences of harm or relational breakdown. As Bernet et al. (2022) define it: "a child's justified contact refusal of a parent, such as due to a history of abuse, neglect, or severely deficient parenting" (p. 6).

Importantly, not all parental flaws constitute grounds for justified estrangement. The concept of the "good enough" parent is relevant here: children may feel disappointed, angry, or disconnected from a parent who is inconsistent or emotionally distant, but unless the parenting reaches a threshold of significant harm, the rejection may not be justified. One of the central challenges for assessors is determining whether the child is rejecting a parent due to genuine protective reasons – or due to distorted perceptions arising from external influence. In cases of justified estrangement, children often report sadness or regret about the lost relationship, but not the intense disdain or moral condemnation typical in PA cases.

Loyalty Conflicts and High-Conflict Dynamics

Another important source of contact refusal can be found in loyalty conflicts, which often emerge in high-conflict separations. In such scenarios, both parents may engage in hostile, coercive, or alienating behaviours. The child is caught in the middle, feeling torn between caregivers and pressured to align with one over the other. These situations may involve:

- Both parents denigrating one another to the child
- Confiding in the child inappropriately
- Encouraging secrecy or emotional allegiance
- Enmeshed relationships with one or both parents

Unlike clear cases of PA, loyalty conflict dynamics may not result in full rejection of either parent, but they can lead to chronic distress, confusion, or behavioural problems. While elements of PA may be present, the dynamic is more mutual, and the child's resistance may shift or fluctuate over time.

Enmeshment

Enmeshment describes a relational pattern in which the boundaries between parent and child are so diffuse that the child's sense of autonomy and independent identity is compromised. Although enmeshment can co-occur with PA, it is not the same thing. In enmeshed relationships, the child often feels responsible for the parent's emotional wellbeing and may suppress their own needs or preferences to maintain closeness.

This dynamic becomes problematic when the child's dependency or identification with one parent leads them to reject the other parent, not because of alienating messages per se, but because the enmeshed bond cannot tolerate divided loyalty. It is essential to differentiate enmeshment from healthy closeness: the former undermines the child's development; the latter supports it.

Parental Gatekeeping

Parental gatekeeping refers to behaviours that limit or control a child's contact with the other parent. Gatekeeping can be protective (e.g., in response to safety concerns) or restrictive (e.g., based on resentment or control). While restrictive gatekeeping can resemble PA, it does not always involve the broader behavioural campaign seen in alienation cases. Gatekeeping may be temporary, reactionary, or context-specific and should not be equated with PA without clear evidence of its impact on the child's beliefs and behaviour.

Hybrid Cases

Perhaps the most complex category is that of hybrid cases, where features of both PA and estrangement are present. These cases often involve a mix of justified and unjustified rejection and may include credible histories of abuse alongside evidence of alienating behaviours. For example:

- A child may have experienced some genuine harm from the targeted parent but is also being manipulated by the aligned parent to reject them more fully than warranted.
- The targeted parent may have engaged in poor or reactive parenting following separation, creating partial but insufficient grounds for rejection.
- Abuse allegations may be used by the alienating parent as a justification for gatekeeping, even when unsubstantiated or exaggerated.

These cases require particularly careful evaluation, as simplistic binaries (alienation *or* abuse) are inadequate. As Bernet et al. (2022) note, hybrid cases were acknowledged with over 80% consensus among experts, but determining what counts as a "legitimate" versus "illegitimate" reason for rejection remains a nuanced and contested task.

Moreover, as Sullivan and Lasley (2010) and Baker et al. (2019) have observed, abused children often continue to show attachment to abusive parents, making behavioural indicators alone an unreliable guide. Understanding hybrid cases demands an appreciation for the interplay of risk, trauma, manipulation, and developmental factors that shape a child's rejection. Current tools for classifying and assessing such cases continue to evolve, and there is a pressing need for greater clarity and consistency in how this category is used in clinical and legal settings.

SUMMARY

This chapter explored the essential task of differentiating parental alienation (PA) from other resist–refuse dynamics that may lead a child to reject a parent. It began by emphasising that, while PA involves the unjustified rejection of a parent due to alienating behaviours, not all contact refusal is pathological or indicative of alienation. The chapter then systematically examined a range of alternative explanations, including developmentally typical resistance, justified estrangement, loyalty conflicts, enmeshment, restrictive gatekeeping, and hybrid cases.

Each of these dynamics was unpacked to show how they differ conceptually and clinically from PA, offering professionals a framework for careful, evidence-informed assessment. Particularly complex are hybrid cases, which combine elements of both PA and legitimate estrangement and demand nuanced clinical and legal judgement. The overarching message is that misapplication of the PA label can obscure other underlying issues and hinder appropriate intervention. Thus, accurate differentiation is both a scientific and ethical imperative.

BIBLIOGRAPHY

Baker, A. J. L., Miller, S., Bernet, W., & Abedayo, T. (2019). The assessment of attitudes and behaviors about physically abused children: A survey of mental health professionals. *Journal of Child and Family Studies, 28*, 3401–3411. https://doi.org/10.1007/s10826-019-01522-5

Bernet, W., Baker, A. J., & Adkins, K. L. (2022). Definitions and terminology regarding child alignments, estrangement, and alienation: A survey of custody evaluators. *Journal of Forensic Sciences, 67*(1), 279–288. https://doi.org/10.1111/1556-4029.14868

Sullivan, R., & Lasley, E. N. (2010). Fear in love: Attachment, abuse, and the developing brain. *Cerebrum: The Dana Forum on Brain Science, 17*.

4

MEASURING PARENTAL ALIENATION

The preceding chapters have established three key foundations. First, parental alienation (PA) can be clearly defined as the unjustified rejection of a parent caused by a pattern of alienating behaviours (Chapter 1). Second, the construct of PA is now underpinned by a growing body of rigorous scientific research, which firmly establishes its validity (Chapter 2). Third, PA is not a "catch-all" explanation for contact problems but must always be carefully distinguished from other resist–refuse dynamics, such as justified estrangement, loyalty conflicts, or hybrid cases (Chapter 3).

Taken together, these insights underscore a critical point: the assessment of PA must be contextual. Alienating behaviours only acquire meaning when their function and outcomes are examined in relation to the child, the targeted parent, and the wider family system. Simply observing contact resistance is not sufficient. Instead, measurement requires a structured, evidence-based framework capable of integrating behavioural data, child outcomes, and contextual considerations.

This chapter examines how PA can be reliably assessed and measured. We begin with the Five-Factor Model proposed by William Bernet, which provides a widely endorsed framework for distinguishing PA from other contact problems. The model outlines five key criteria that must be met in order to establish PA, ranging from the presence of a previously positive parent–child relationship to evidence of alienating behaviours and the absence of

DOI: 10.4324/9781003630944-6

legitimate reasons for rejection. We then turn to the tools currently available for measuring both alienating behaviours (the process) and the child's rejection of the targeted parent (the outcome). Together, these approaches provide a systematic basis for identifying PA, differentiating it from other dynamics, and informing appropriate clinical and legal responses.

THE FIVE-FACTOR MODEL OF PARENTAL ALIENATION

William Bernet's Five-Factor Model is one of the most widely recognised frameworks for assessing whether a child's resistance or refusal of contact constitutes parental alienation (PA). Building on earlier four-factor models, it introduces an additional focus on the child's rejection itself, creating a more complete and systematic structure for distinguishing PA from other resist–refuse dynamics, such as justified estrangement, loyalty conflicts, or hybrid cases (Bernet & Greenhill, 2022; Morrison & Ring, 2023).

The model requires evaluators to consider multiple dimensions of the family system, the child, the targeted parent, the aligned (alienating) parent, and the history of relationships, rather than relying on any single indicator. Each factor must be examined in depth, with particular attention to context, proportionality, and corroborated evidence. Together, the five factors offer a comprehensive guide for determining whether rejection reflects alienation.

Factor One: Contact Resistance or Refusal

The model begins with the most visible symptom: the child's rejection or resistance to contact with one parent. This is a necessary but not sufficient condition for PA. A wide range of factors may explain contact refusal (see Chapter 3), including abuse, estrangement, or developmental issues. What distinguishes PA is that the child's rejection is frequent, consistent, and persistent, and appears out of proportion to anything the rejected parent has done.

Research demonstrates that even physically abused children often seek to maintain relationships with abusive parents, displaying attachment-seeking rather than attachment-breaking behaviours (Baker et al., 2019). In contrast, alienated children may exhibit total rejection, contempt, or fear towards a safe and "good enough" parent. Assessing the severity and persistence of the rejection is, therefore, the first step in identifying PA.

Factor Two: Prior Positive Relationship with the Rejected Parent

Central to the model is whether the child once shared a healthy and loving relationship with the now-rejected parent. A sudden shift from warmth and affection to hostility and rejection, absent intervening abuse or neglect, is a strong indicator of alienation.

Evidence of a prior positive bond may include photographs, cards, videos, school reports, witness testimony, or therapist notes documenting affection, involvement, and responsiveness. Importantly, this factor distinguishes PA from long-standing estrangement or disrupted attachment histories. If the parent–child relationship was consistently marginal or conflicted, then alienation may not be the correct framework. Conversely, when a previously secure relationship is abruptly severed following separation, alienation becomes the more likely explanation.

Factor Three: Absence of Abuse, Neglect, or Seriously Deficient Parenting

The third factor requires establishing that the rejected parent has not engaged in behaviours that reasonably justify rejection. This means excluding substantiated abuse, neglect, or significant parenting failures as the basis of the child's hostility.

Assessment should draw on multiple, objective sources, such as child protection records, court findings, or independent clinical evaluations. Allegations must be scrutinised for consistency and timing, as false or exaggerated claims are common in alienation contexts. A critical task here is proportionality: does the intensity of the child's rejection correspond to the actual parenting they experienced? If the rejection is excessive or illogical in light of the parent's behaviour, PA is a strong possibility.

Hybrid cases complicate this factor, as a parent may have displayed some deficits (e.g., poor conflict management, emotional withdrawal) without reaching a threshold that would normally cause total rejection. In such cases, alienating behaviours by the favoured parent may be amplifying and distorting the child's perceptions.

Factor Four: Alienating Parent's Behaviours

The fourth factor examines the behaviours of the aligned or favoured parent. Alienation is rarely accidental; it typically involves a pattern of repeated, intentional behaviours designed to undermine the child's relationship with the other parent. Bernet has catalogued 17 common alienating behaviours (see Chapter 1), ranging from overt denigration to more subtle forms of manipulation. These include:

- Badmouthing or blaming the targeted parent.
- Limiting contact or interfering with communication.
- Withholding important information.
- Encouraging secrecy or disobedience.
- Creating the impression the targeted parent is dangerous or unloving.
- Rewarding rejection or punishing affection.
- Encouraging the child to choose sides.

- Using inappropriate confidences or adult topics.
- Making false allegations of abuse.
- Enlisting others to reinforce rejection.

These behaviours may be direct (e.g., explicit denigration) or indirect (e.g., non-verbal disapproval when the child mentions the other parent). Acts of omission are also significant, such as failing to correct others' negative comments about the targeted parent. Crucially, a pattern of multiple behaviours over time must be present to indicate alienation.

Factor Five: Child's Behavioural Manifestations

The final factor looks at the child's own behaviours and attitudes towards the targeted parent. Bernet identified eight key manifestations that are distinctive to alienated children:

1. Campaign of denigration – ongoing hostility towards the rejected parent.
2. Frivolous rationalisations – trivial or illogical reasons for rejection.
3. Lack of ambivalence – splitting one parent as "all good" and the other as "all bad."
4. Independent thinker phenomenon – insisting rejection is their own decision.
5. Reflexive support – automatic siding with the favoured parent.
6. Borrowed scenarios – repeating adult phrases or stories they could not know.
7. Lack of guilt or remorse – no empathy for the rejected parent's pain.
8. Spread of animosity – hostility extends to the targeted parent's family, friends, and even pets.

These signs are rarely present in cases of justified estrangement. For example, estranged children may express sadness or regret about losing a parent, whereas alienated children often display contempt or indifference.

The Value of the Five-Factor Model

Taken together, the Five-Factor Model provides a structured, evidence-based framework for distinguishing PA from other forms of contact refusal. Its strength lies in integrating multiple perspectives: the child's behaviour, the parent's history, the presence of alienating behaviours, and the overall family context. It avoids simplistic attributions (e.g., "the child is resisting, therefore it must be PA") and instead demands a comprehensive, contextualised analysis.

The model has been validated in empirical research and widely endorsed by professionals across disciplines. It is particularly valuable in high-conflict custody disputes, where careful differentiation between alienation, estrangement, and hybrid cases is essential to avoid misapplication.

MEASURING ALIENATING BEHAVIOURS AND CHILD REJECTION

With increasing conceptual clarity about what PA is and how it manifests, scholars have developed a range of measures to assess both the processes that produce alienation (Parental Alienating Behaviours, or PABs) and the outcomes (the child's rejection or resistance towards a parent). This development challenges one of the common myths repeated in critical discourse, that no reliable or valid measures of PA exist (Freeman, 2020). In fact, the field now has a variety of instruments, many with strong psychometric properties and preliminary validation across different cultural contexts.

Much like the measurement landscape in domestic violence and abuse research, the current status of PA measurement can be described as pluralistic but robust (Bowen, 2011). Several tools exist, each with their strengths and limitations, offering professionals multiple entry points into assessment depending on the nature of the case and the information required.

Measures of Parental Alienating Behaviours (PABs)

These instruments aim to capture the strategies used by the alienating parent to undermine the child's relationship with the targeted parent:

- Rowlands Parental Alienation Scale (RPAS; Rowlands, 2019, 2020): A targeted measure focusing on specific alienating behaviours, capturing their presence, frequency, and severity. This measure is useful in identifying patterns of manipulation and distinguishing them from more benign family conflict behaviours.
- Parental Alienation Questionnaire (PAQ; Sîrbu et al., 2021): A self-report tool designed to assess alienating behaviours from the perspective of the targeted parent. It includes items on denigration, obstruction of contact, and manipulation, providing an overview of how such behaviours are experienced.
- ZICAP II (Zicavo Martínez et al., 2021): Developed and validated in Chile, this instrument assesses PABs within Latin American cultural contexts. Its emergence illustrates the international recognition of PA and the need for culturally adaptable measurement tools.
- A new 30-Item PAB Scale (Varvei & Harman, 2025): This measure was developed to assess a wide range of parental alienating behaviours beyond simple denigration, including guilt induction, loyalty conflicts, and restriction of time with the targeted parent. Participants rate 30 behaviours separately for mothers and fathers, with examples such as

"My mother made me feel guilty if I enjoyed time with my father" and "My mother encouraged me to spend less time with my father."

Together, these measures highlight the multi-dimensional nature of PABs and the importance of distinguishing deliberate alienating practices from more ambiguous conflict behaviours.

Measures of Child Rejection and Acceptance

The outcome of PA is best captured through instruments that assess the child's attitudes, behaviours, and alignment with each parent. These tools focus on how alienating behaviours manifest in the child's relational stance.

- Parental Acceptance-Rejection Questionnaire (PARQ; Rohner & Ali, 2020): A widely validated tool originally designed to assess perceived parental warmth and rejection. It has been adapted in PA research to capture how children internalise alienating narratives and display rejection.
- Parental Alienation Scale (PAS; Baker): A self-report measure for targeted parents, assessing both alienating behaviours and child outcomes, such as hostility, denigration, and withdrawal. It provides a quantitative indication of the severity of alienation.
- Child Affected by Parental Relationship Distress (CAPRD; DSM-5): Although not a specific instrument, CAPRD provides a recognised clinical category for children exhibiting psychological distress due to disrupted parental relationships, including PA dynamics. It offers a framework for considering PA within established diagnostic systems.
- Observational Measures: Parent–Child Interaction Assessment-II (PCIA-II) and the Dyadic Parent–Child Interaction Coding System (DPICS) observational protocols provide objective data on child–parent interactions, highlighting both avoidance and acceptance behaviours. These tools are particularly valuable for capturing discrepancies between what children say and how they behave in real time.

Broader Evaluations and Expert Assessments

Beyond structured instruments, expert evaluations remain central in PA assessment. These typically involve interviews with all family members, collateral contacts (teachers, extended family), and review of documents such as school records, medical notes, or prior court findings. While more resource-intensive, expert evaluations provide the contextual depth often required in complex or hybrid cases.

CHALLENGES IN ASSESSING PARENTAL ALIENATION

Although a growing range of measurement tools now exist, evaluating parental alienation (PA) in practice remains a complex and often contentious task. Several challenges stand out.

First, many alienating behaviours are subtle, indirect, or covert, making them difficult to capture through straightforward observation or self-report. Non-verbal cues, omissions, or manipulation framed as concern for the child can be easily missed, potentially leading to either an underestimation or an over-interpretation of the problem.

Second, the limitations of self-report instruments must be acknowledged. Targeted parents, often distressed, may unintentionally exaggerate their perceptions of alienating behaviours, while alienating parents are likely to minimise or deny their actions. Alienated children themselves may be so aligned with the favoured parent that they repeat distorted narratives as if they were their own, further complicating accurate assessment.

Third, confounding variables within family systems, such as pre-existing high conflict, parental psychopathology, or histories of poor relationship quality, can obscure the distinction between alienation and other causes of contact resistance. Assessors must take care to separate the influence of these factors from the specific contribution of alienating behaviours.

Despite these difficulties, precise and reliable assessment is essential. However, only by using a multi-method, evidence-based approach, integrating interviews, observations, psychometrics, and collateral data, can professionals mitigate bias, contextualise findings, and ensure that decisions about children's welfare are grounded in an accurate understanding of the family dynamics.

Core Elements of Assessment

When undertaking an evaluation of suspected PA, professionals should consider several core elements:

- Relationship history: The quality of the child's relationship with each parent prior to separation, as well as the wider family dynamics, including extended family and patterns of conflict.
- The child's behaviours: Unexplained hostility, a lack of ambivalence, or the use of language that appears borrowed from the aligned parent may be indicators of alienation.
- The alienating parent's actions: Consistent denigration, obstruction of contact, or inducement of loyalty are key signals of alienating behaviours.
- The targeted parent's responses: Assessing the psychological and emotional impact on the rejected parent provides insight into both the severity of the alienation and its consequences for family functioning.

These dimensions should not be examined in isolation but as interacting features of a dynamic system.

Techniques for Identifying Manifestations in Children

Professionals have several techniques at their disposal when determining whether a child's rejection is indicative of alienation:

- Interviews: One-to-one interviews with the child can uncover their perceptions, reasons for resistance, and whether these appear to be independently formed or externally influenced.
- Observations: Structured observations of the child with each parent, across different contexts such as home, school, or clinic, can highlight inconsistencies in behaviour and relational comfort.
- Psychological testing: Standardised instruments may reveal signs of emotional manipulation, anxiety, or distorted cognitions about a parent.
- Collateral information: Data from schools, medical professionals, or extended family can provide additional perspectives, although evaluators must remain cautious about potential institutional or systemic reinforcement of alienation.
- Developmental sensitivity: A child's age and stage of development shape how they express loyalty, fear, or rejection. Assessments must be tailored accordingly.
- Cultural and contextual awareness: Family practices, cultural expectations, and environmental stressors can influence how alienation manifests, and must be accounted for when interpreting findings.
- Repeated assessments: Because alienation is not static but a progressive process, assessments conducted at multiple time points can provide a more reliable picture of how dynamics evolve.

SUMMARY

The assessment of parental alienation requires a holistic and methodologically rigorous approach, one that balances sensitivity to subtle dynamics with the demand for robust evidence. By integrating diverse tools and perspectives, and by situating behaviours in their relational and cultural context, practitioners can make well-grounded distinctions between alienation, estrangement, and other forms of resist–refuse dynamics. This is critical not only for academic precision but, more importantly, for ensuring that legal and clinical interventions genuinely serve the best interests of children and families.

BIBLIOGRAPHY

Baker, A. J. L., Miller, S., Bernet, W., & Abedayo, T. (2019). The assessment of attitudes and behaviors about physically abused children: A survey of mental health professionals. *Journal of Child and Family Studies*, *28*, 3401–3411. https://doi.org/10.1007/s10826-019-01522-5

Bernet, W., & Greenhill, L. L. (2022). The five-factor model for the diagnosis of parental alienation. *Journal of the American Academy of Child & Adolescent Psychiatry, 61*, 591–594. https://doi.org/10.1016/j.jaac.2021.11.026

Bowen, E. (2011). An overview of partner violence risk assessment and the potential role of female victim risk appraisals. *Aggression and Violent Behavior, 16*, 214–226. https://doi.org/10.1016/j.avb.2011.02.007

Eyberg, S. M., Nelson, M. M., Duke, M., & Boggs, S. R. (2005). *Manual for the Dyadic parent–child Interaction coding system* (3rd ed.). Gainesville, FL: PCIT International.

Freeman, B. (2020). The psychosocial assessment of contact refusal. In D. Lorandos & W. Bernet (Eds.), *Parental alienation – science and law* (pp. 44–81). Charles C Thomas Publisher, Ltd.

Holigrocki, R. J., Kaminski, P. L., & Frieswyk, S. H. (2002). *Parent-child interaction assessment II (PCIA-II): Directions for administration*. Unpublished manuscript. Manuscript will be mailed upon request. Dr. Holigrocki or Dr. Kaminski for a copy (Update of PCIA Tech. Rep. No. 99-1046. Topeka, KS: Child and Family Center, The Menninger Clinic).

Morrison, S. L., & Ring, R. (2023). Reliability of the five-factor model for determining parental alienation. *The American Journal of Family Therapy, 51*, 580–598. https://doi.org/10.1080/01926187.2021.2021831

Rohner, R. P., & Ali, S. (2020). Parental acceptance-rejection questionnaire (PARQ). In *Encyclopedia of personality and individual differences*. Springer. https://doi.org/10.1007/978-3-319-24612-3_56

Rowlands, G. A. (2019). Parental alienation: A measurement tool. *Divorce & Remarriage, 60*, 316–331. https://doi.org/10.1080/10502556.2018.1546031

Rowlands, G. A. (2020). Parental alienation: A measurement tool confirmatory analysis validation study. *Journal of Divorce and Remarriage, 61*, 127–147. https://doi.org/10.1080/10502556.2019.1627162

Sîrbu, A. G., Vintilă, M., Tisu, L., Stefănut, A. M., Tudorel, O. I., Măguran, B., & Toma, R. A. (2021). Parental alienation – development and validation of a behavioral anchor scale. *Sustainability, 13*, 1–18. https://doi.org/2071-1050/13/1/316

Varavei, H., & Harman, J. J. (2025). At what point does a behavior become child abuse? A closer look at the chronicity of child maltreatment and demographic factors. *International Journal on Child Maltreatment: Research, Policy and Practice, 8*, 1–41. https://doi.org/10.1007/s42448-025-00227-1

Zicavo Martínez, N., Rey Clericus, R., & Ponce, L. (2021). ZICAP II scale: Parental alienation assessment in 9 to 15 years-old children of separated parents in Chile. *Ciencias Psicológicas, 15*. https://doi.org/10.22235/cp.v15i1.2159

5

PREVALENCE

Having clarified in earlier chapters what parental alienation (PA) is, how it differs from other resist–refuse dynamics, and how it can be measured through both behaviours and outcomes, we are now in a position to ask a crucial question: *how widespread is the problem?* Understanding prevalence is essential for appreciating the scale of the issue, shaping professional awareness, and informing the allocation of legal, clinical, and policy resources. With clearer definitions and validated tools, researchers can more accurately identify cases of PA and parental alienating behaviours (PABs), allowing us to move beyond anecdotal accounts and contested assumptions to an evidence-informed estimate of how many children and families are affected.

PREVALENCE OF ALIENATING BEHAVIOURS

Attempts to estimate how common parental alienating behaviours (PABs) are have produced varied results, largely because of differences in methods and sampling. Much of the early work relied on clinical or legal samples, which, while important, tend to overrepresent high-conflict families. For example, Clawar and Rivlin (1991, 2013) documented alienating behaviours in the majority of custody-dispute cases they examined.

In order to capture prevalence beyond high-conflict samples, researchers have increasingly turned to population-based data. Harman et al. (2016)

DOI: 10.4324/9781003630944-7

used a representative poll in North Carolina and found that 13.4 percent of parents had been subjected to alienating behaviours. This line of work was extended in a nationally representative online survey of parents in the United States and Canada, which reported that 35.5 percent of US parents and 32 percent of Canadian parents described experiences consistent with exposure to PABs (Harman et al., 2019). Comparable figures have now emerged from the United Kingdom. In a representative study of 1,005 separated or divorced parents, between 39 and 59 percent reported experiencing PABs, with 36.5 percent identified as non-reciprocating targeted parents (Hine et al., 2025a).

Taken together, these studies suggest that alienating behaviours are not rare; rather, a substantial minority of separated or divorced parents report being exposed to them. At the same time, variation in reported prevalence is strongly shaped by methodological decisions, particularly whether data come from clinical samples, which yield higher rates, or general population samples, which provide a more conservative estimate. Moreover, most of this research is currently limited to North America and the UK, leaving significant gaps in our understanding of how widespread these behaviours are in other cultural contexts.

PREVALENCE OF PARENTAL ALIENATION

While exposure to PABs is relatively common, the outcome of parental alienation (PA) appears to be less frequent and more complex to establish. This reflects the importance of distinguishing alienation from justified estrangement and situating rejection within the broader family context.

Representative studies provide the clearest data. In their US–Canada survey, Harman et al. (2019) found that while one in three parents reported exposure to PABs, only 6.7 percent of separated or divorced parents believed their children were moderately to severely alienated. This equated to roughly 1.3 percent of the national population in the United States. Earlier estimates, often based on high-conflict samples, tended to be higher. For instance, Bernet et al. (2010) and Warshak (2015) estimated that between 20 and 25 percent of children in high-conflict divorces experience some level of alienation.

More recent UK evidence underscores the importance of contextual criteria. In the representative survey of 1,005 parents, while 39 to 59 percent reported exposure to PABs, only 3.5 percent met criteria for PA when contextual features such as a prior positive parent–child relationship were considered. Similarly, although nearly all parents reported some alienation-type behaviours in their children (96.7 percent), only 2.9 percent met the stricter threshold for PA as an outcome (Hine et al., 2025b).

These findings highlight a consistent pattern: PABs are widespread, but PA is much less common when robust definitions and contextualised assessment models, such as Bernet's Five-Factor Model, are applied. The discrepancy between the prevalence of behaviours and the outcome underscores the danger of conflating exposure to PABs with entrenched alienation. Distinguishing between these levels is critical for research, practice, and policy.

TRANSLATING PREVALENCE RATES INTO POPULATION ESTIMATES

The prevalence figures from representative studies in the United Kingdom (Hine et al., 2025b) allow us to make approximate projections of how many families might be affected in different national contexts. If the UK rates, 39 to 59 percent of separated or divorced parents reporting exposure to parental alienating behaviours (PABs), and 3.5 percent of children meeting criteria for parental alienation (PA) outcomes when contextual factors are applied, were observed elsewhere, this would translate into millions of affected families worldwide. The table below applies these percentages to available estimates of separated or divorced parent populations in the United States, Canada, the United Kingdom, and Australia. For countries such as India, China, Brazil, and Spain, where reliable statistics on separated or divorced parents with children are lacking, figures cannot yet be calculated with any degree of confidence.

Country	*Estimate of Separated/Divorced Parents**	*39–59% of those → Estimated Exposure to PABs*	*3.5% of those → Estimated Meeting PA Criteria*
United States	~30–40 million	≈11.7–23.6 million	≈1.05–1.40 million
Canada	~4–6 million	≈1.56–3.54 million	≈0.14–0.21 million
United Kingdom	~6–8 million	≈2.34–4.72 million	≈0.21–0.28 million
Australia	~2–3 million	≈0.78–1.77 million	≈0.07–0.11 million

Caveats and Limitations

It is crucial to treat these figures as illustrative rather than definitive. First, they depend on the accuracy of national statistics regarding the number of separated or divorced parents, which vary in quality and completeness across countries. Many existing figures conflate all divorces (including childless marriages) or fail to capture separations outside of formal legal processes, both of which can distort prevalence estimates. Second, applying UK prevalence rates to other nations assumes that alienating behaviours and alienation outcomes occur at similar frequencies across very different cultural, social, and legal contexts. This is unlikely to be the case: norms around parenting, custody arrangements, and conflict resolution vary substantially worldwide. Finally, the UK data themselves highlight how prevalence estimates are highly sensitive to definitional and methodological choices, particularly whether contextual criteria (such as a prior positive parent–child relationship) are included.

SUMMARY

This chapter explored what is currently known about the prevalence of PABs and PA. Research consistently shows that PABs are widespread in separated and divorced families, though estimates vary depending on methodology. Early studies of high-conflict clinical samples reported very high rates, while more recent population-based surveys in the United States, Canada, and the United Kingdom suggest that roughly one-third to one-half of separated parents report exposure to PABs. By contrast, the outcome of PA, where a child unjustifiably rejects a parent and manifests this in their behaviour, is far less common. US and Canadian data suggest that around 6 to 7 percent of separated parents believe their children are moderately to severely alienated, while UK research using contextual criteria has produced lower figures of around 3.5 percent. These findings underscore an important distinction: alienating behaviours are frequently present, but entrenched alienation is less prevalent when carefully defined.

To illustrate the potential scale of the issue, UK prevalence rates were applied to separated and divorced parent populations in several Western countries, suggesting that millions of families are likely affected. However, such estimates must be treated with caution. Reliable figures on separated parents are not consistently available, and applying UK rates across countries with different cultural, legal, and social contexts risks oversimplification. What is clear is that alienating behaviours are a significant issue across separated families, yet more cross-cultural, methodologically rigorous research is needed to refine global prevalence estimates and ensure they are useful for clinical, legal, and policy responses.

BIBLIOGRAPHY

Bernet, W., von Boch-Galhau, W., Baker, A. J. L., & Morrison, S. L. (2010). Parental alienation, DSM-V, and ICD-11. *The American Journal of Family Therapy*, *38*(2), 76–187. https://doi.org/10.1080/01926180903586583

Clawar, S. S., & Rivlin, B. V. (1991). *Children held hostage: Dealing with programmed and brainwashed children*. American Bar Association Press.

Clawar, S. S., & Rivlin, B. V. (2013). *Children held hostage: Identifying brainwashed children, presenting a case, and crafting solutions*. American Bar Association Press.

Harman, J. J., Leder-Elder, S., & Biringen, Z. (2016). Prevalence of parental alienation drawn from a representative poll. *Children and Youth Services Review*, *66*, 62–66. https://doi.org/10.1016/j.childyouth.2016.04.021

Harman, J. J., Leder-Elder, S., & Biringen, Z. (2019). Prevalence of adults who are the targets of parental alienating behaviors and their impact. *Children and Youth Services Review*, *106*, 104471. https://doi.org/10.1016/j.childyouth.2019.104471

Hine, B. A., Harman, J. J., Leder-Elder, S., & Bates, E. A. (2025a). Examining the prevalence and impact of parental alienating behaviors (PABs) in separated parents in the United Kingdom. *Journal of Family Violence*. https://doi.org/10.1007/s10896-025-00910-4

Hine, B. A., Harman, J. J., Leder-Elder, S., & Bates, E. A. (2025b). *Examining the prevalence and impact of parental alienating behaviors (PABs) in adults aged 18–25 years in the United Kingdom.* Manuscript Under Review.

Warshak, R. (2015). Parental alienation: Overview, management, intervention, and practice tips. *Journal of the American Academy of Matrimonial Lawyers, 28*, 181.

PART 2

WHY DOES IT HAPPEN?

6

UNDERSTANDING ALIENATING PARENTS

Parental Alienation is enacted, consciously or unconsciously, by individuals whose behaviours and motivations demand close scrutiny. This chapter turns our attention to the perpetrators of alienation: those who systematically undermine a child's relationship with the other parent. While the mechanisms of alienation are often subtle, complex, and embedded within wider relational dynamics, they are not random. Understanding who these individuals are, what drives their behaviours, and how they operate, emotionally, psychologically, and socially, is essential for recognising the patterns that lead to alienation. Drawing on available research and theory, this chapter maps the characteristics commonly found in perpetrators, including tendencies towards coercive control, psychological vulnerability, and distorted relational needs. By focusing first on the behaviours and profiles of those who alienate, we lay the foundation for the following chapters, which will explore the theoretical frameworks, particularly attachment theory and coercive control, that explain why these behaviours emerge and persist.

UNWITTING AND SITUATIONAL ALIENATORS: THE MILD END OF THE SPECTRUM

In less severe cases of parental alienation, alienating behaviours often arise from poor boundaries, emotional enmeshment, unresolved conflict, or

DOI: 10.4324/9781003630944-9

inadequate coping mechanisms. These parents may not fully comprehend the consequences of their actions, and their intent is not to harm but to manage their own distress.

- *Unresolved Emotional Issues*: These parents may be consumed by feelings of betrayal, hurt, or humiliation following separation. They might over-share their distress with the child, unconsciously recruit them as emotional allies, or foster resentment towards the targeted parent under the guise of "truth-telling." The unresolved anger, betrayal, or humiliation from the adult relationship can thus drive a parent to co-opt the child as a vehicle for revenge, with the child then becoming the battleground upon which unresolved grievances are played out. Such dynamics may be particularly pronounced in cases where the alienating parent perceives the end of the relationship as unjust or humiliating, fuelling a desire to "punish" the former partner by depriving them of a parental role.
- *Inadequate Coping Skills*: These contribute significantly to alienating behaviour. Some parents, overwhelmed by the emotional and logistical demands of separation, resort to manipulation, control, and exclusion as methods of regaining psychological stability. Emotional overwhelm, poor stress tolerance, and fear of losing the child can drive behaviour that prioritises the alienating parent's needs over the child's wellbeing. Disclosure of adult material, passive-aggressive scheduling, or subtle discouragement of contact may occur with little awareness of the harm caused. As such, these parents may not understand the impact of their actions, particularly in early-stage alienation, and may benefit from psychoeducation and supportive therapeutic intervention. However, without recognition of harm and sustained intervention, these behaviours can become entrenched.
- *Perceived Threats and Overprotection*: In some cases, the alienating parent may genuinely believe they are protecting the child from harm. This belief may arise from past experiences of abuse, distorted perceptions of the other parent, or misinformation perpetuated by legal or professional actors. While protective instincts are not inherently pathological, they become problematic when based on exaggerated, false, or uncorroborated claims that lead to unjustified estrangement. The moral certainty with which these parents act often makes intervention difficult, as they interpret professional concern as an attack rather than a safeguard.

  This perceived threat framework intersects with coercive control (see Chapter 9). As in cases of intimate partner violence, alienating parents may seek to reassert control post-separation through the child. The more the other parent attempts to assert their role, the more aggressively the alienator reacts, escalating behaviours that aim to exclude and discredit.

In this way, the child becomes both shield and weapon, used to neutralise the threat of the other parent's continued presence.
- *Intergenerational Transmission*: Parents who themselves experienced alienation, emotional neglect, or unhealthy family enmeshment may unconsciously replicate those patterns. A history of enmeshment, emotional cut-offs, or parental triangulation may normalise maladaptive patterns that are then unconsciously replicated. Without insight or therapeutic support, they may regard their behaviours as normative or justified, repeating the trauma that shaped their own developmental trajectory.

Situational alienators are often responsive to psychoeducation, structured parenting interventions, and therapeutic support. With clear judicial expectations and early intervention, many can modify their behaviours and restore healthier family dynamics.

PATHOLOGICALLY DRIVEN ALIENATORS: THE MODERATE TO SEVERE END

At the more entrenched end of the spectrum are individuals whose alienating behaviours are underpinned by significant personality pathology, unresolved trauma, or characterological rigidity. These alienators typically lack insight, deny personal responsibility, and are resistant to change, even when faced with evidence of harm.

- *Narcissistic Personality Traits*: Narcissistic Personality Disorder (NPD) is typified by grandiosity, a fragile self-concept, and an absence of empathy. In the context of parental alienation, individuals with narcissistic traits often perceive their children not as independent agents with their own needs but as extensions of their own self-image. The targeted parent, particularly if perceived as a threat to the alienator's superiority or identity, becomes a psychological enemy to be eliminated. The alienating parent may expect the child to mirror their negative views, reinforcing a shared narrative of vilification that bolsters their self-esteem. Empirical research suggests that narcissistically aligned alienating parents are often skilled at manipulating perceptions, both of the child and of professionals, in order to maintain control over the family narrative.
- *Borderline Personality Traits*: Borderline Personality Disorder (BPD) presents another clinical profile strongly associated with alienating behaviours. Marked by emotional dysregulation, a pervasive fear of abandonment, and interpersonal instability, individuals with BPD may experience the post-separation parenting dynamic as a site of existential threat. To mitigate perceived abandonment by the child, the alienating parent may engage in coercive bonding strategies, fostering dependence,

emotional enmeshment, and rejection of the other parent. This dynamic can rapidly evolve into a pattern where the child's loyalty becomes both currency and proof of love, and the targeted parent is cast as a dangerous interloper.

- *Histrionic Personality Traits*: Histrionic Personality Disorder (HPD), though less commonly discussed in the context of parental alienation, could also play a notable role. Individuals with HPD often exhibit dramatic emotionality, attention-seeking behaviour, and relational instability. In family systems, they may manufacture or exaggerate distress to elicit sympathy, leveraging the child's emotional responsiveness to strengthen the alliance. Their narratives of victimisation may be compelling to courts and professionals, often masking the manipulative dynamics beneath. Importantly, their tendency to idealise and devalue others can contribute to extreme polarisation between the parents in the child's mind.
- *The Dark Triad*: Some severe alienators exhibit traits associated with the Dark Triad – *narcissism*, *Machiavellianism*, and *psychopathy*. The Dark Triad thus offers a dimensional model for understanding manipulative tendencies often found in more severe alienators. Machiavellian traits (manipulativeness, strategic deception) can manifest in the calculated undermining of the other parent's role, while psychopathic traits (callousness, lack of remorse) may account for the absence of guilt and the instrumental use of the child. While not all alienating parents meet clinical thresholds for these traits, their presence in moderate to severe cases is well documented, especially when behaviours escalate despite judicial or therapeutic intervention.

In these cases, alienation is not simply a byproduct of distress or confusion; the behaviours are rigid, persistent, and resistant to corrective input. As research increasingly demonstrates, these cases require a child protection framework, often including removal from the alienating parent's care, structured reunification programmes, and legal sanctions to prevent ongoing harm.

MMPI-2 Profiles and the Psychological Portrait of Alienating Parents

As the field matures, research increasingly emphasises the need for empirically validated tools to distinguish between alienating and non-alienating parents. One of the most informative psychological instruments in this context is the Minnesota Multiphasic Personality Inventory-2 (MMPI-2). Two key studies by Roma and colleagues (2021, 2022) have significantly advanced our understanding of how alienating parents, particularly mothers, present on psychometric assessment, highlighting both overt and covert dimensions of their psychological functioning.

In the first study, the researchers analysed the MMPI-2 results of mothers who had been identified as alienating their children. The findings revealed a characteristic pattern of:

- Elevated scores in moral virtue and extraversion, indicating a tendency to present oneself in an overly favourable, socially desirable light.
- Increased interpersonal vulnerability and emotional dysregulation, reflecting heightened sensitivity to relational stressors.
- Unsuccessful self-representation, suggesting difficulty maintaining a coherent and stable self-concept, especially under stress.

This psychometric profile reflects a defensive psychological posture, in which surface-level sociability and idealised self-image mask underlying emotional instability and dependency needs. These patterns align closely with clinical observations of alienating parents who appear cooperative and morally grounded to professionals, yet manipulate the child and undermine the other parent through covert tactics.

The second study extended this analysis by comparing MMPI-2 profiles of 41 couples involved in PA to 39 control couples engaged in custody disputes without alienation. This comparative design revealed several critical distinctions:

- Alienating mothers were found to exhibit a "faking-good" defensive profile, marked by denial of hostile or negative impulses, projection of blame onto others, and high interpersonal sensitivity. This profile illustrates an effort to appear well-adjusted and morally correct while avoiding responsibility for negative behaviour.
- Targeted fathers, by contrast, tended to present profiles consistent with chronic depressive states, social withdrawal, and interpersonal conflict, suggesting a pattern of internalised distress and prolonged psychological burden consistent with the experience of being alienated from a child.

Together, these studies provide a preliminary model for the psychological assessment of alienating parents, offering empirical support for patterns that have long been observed clinically. They reinforce the notion that alienating behaviour is not merely situational or reactive but often reflects underlying personality organisation characterised by defensiveness, projection, and impaired emotional regulation. These patterns can make alienating parents particularly resistant to therapeutic intervention and prone to manipulation of professionals and systems of authority.

The forensic implications are considerable. MMPI-2 assessments can:

- Assist in the differentiation between alienation and justified estrangement.

- Provide a valid, structured insight into defensive and maladaptive traits.
- Inform intervention planning, especially when assessing amenability to change.
- Support legal decision-making around custody and contact, particularly in high-conflict or ambiguous cases.

Importantly, these findings also highlight the necessity for clinicians and legal professionals to approach self-report and in-court behaviour with a critical lens. Alienating parents may construct persuasive narratives of victimhood or virtue that diverge significantly from the psychological realities revealed through standardised assessment.

THE ROLE OF CUSTODIAL STATUS AND GENDER

While custodial parents often have more opportunity to enact alienating behaviours due to proximity and control, alienation is not limited to custodial arrangements, nor is it gender-specific. Fathers and mothers alienate at comparable rates, and non-custodial alienators can be equally effective, especially when supported by extended family, new partners, or uncritical professionals.

The key factor is not who the parent is but how they behave and why, and whether they are unaware and distressed or entitled and calculating. Understanding intent, psychological structure, and patterns of behaviours is therefore essential in differentiating appropriate interventions, and in determining the line between support and protection.

UNDERSTANDING WITHOUT BLAME

As we have and will continue to examine the complex behaviours associated with parental alienation, particularly those of the alienating parent, it is vital to adopt a stance of informed understanding rather than blame. The purpose of this analysis is not to condemn, diagnose, or stigmatise but to deepen our comprehension of the psychological and relational processes at play, so that interventions can be targeted, humane, and effective.

The traits and dynamics often discussed in this context, such as narcissism, manipulation, entitlement, or emotional coercion, can seem confronting. However, it is essential to recognise that not all individuals exhibiting such traits will engage in alienating behaviours, and where they do, those behaviours may be shaped by unresolved trauma, fear of abandonment, identity fragility, or a deep sense of relational threat. Pathology is rarely the whole story. The alienating parent may also be a person in psychological distress, operating from learned defences or internalised relational scripts shaped by earlier life experiences.

Understanding these drivers allows professionals to move beyond simplistic labels and instead respond with clinical curiosity and therapeutic precision. It enables a shift from punitive thinking towards contextualised intervention; approaches that take into account the emotional needs, attachment strategies, and coping mechanisms of all family members.

This does not mean minimising harm. Alienating behaviours can be emotionally abusive, and their impact on children is often profound. But recognising that these behaviours may arise from maladaptive attempts to manage loss, powerlessness, or emotional threat opens up space for more compassionate, systemic intervention – ones that seek not only to stop the behaviour but also to transform the relational dynamics beneath it.

Ultimately, addressing parental alienation effectively requires us to resist polarised thinking. Interventions must be tailored to the unique psychological landscape of each family, recognising that alienation exists on a continuum, and that rigid, one-size-fits-all solutions rarely succeed. A stance of empathy, balanced with clear boundaries and a firm commitment to the child's best interests, is not only ethically necessary but also practically essential.

As we continue through this book, the goal remains clear: to illuminate the behaviours without vilifying the individuals, to identify patterns without erasing complexity, and to support healing that includes, rather than excludes, all members of the family system.

BIBLIOGRAPHY

Darnall, D. C. (2013). Mild cases of parental alienation. In D. Lorandos, W. Bernet, & S. R. Sauber (Eds.), *Parental alienation: The handbook for mental health and legal professionals* (pp. 74–96). Charles C Thomas Publisher, Ltd.

Gilbar, O., Taft, C., & Dekel, R. (2020). Male intimate partner violence: Examining the roles of childhood trauma, PTSD symptoms, and dominance. *Journal of Family Psychology*, *34*, 1004–1013. https://doi.org/10.1037/fam0000669

Harman, J. J., Maniotes, C. R., & Grubb, C. (2021). Power dynamics in families affected by parental alienation. *Personal Relationships*. https://doi.org/10.1111/pere.12392

Lorandos, D., Bernet, W., & Sauber, S. R. (2013). *Parental alienation: The handbook for mental health and legal professionals* (Vol. 1116). Charles C Thomas Publisher, Ltd.

Palmieri, A., Visintainer, V., Toffanin, L., & Picone, V. C. (2024). Role of narcissism in parental alienation phenomenon. A narrative review. *Rivista di psichiatria*, *59*, 45–51. https://doi.org/10.1708/4259.42357

Roma, P., Marchetti, D., Mazza, C., Burla, F., & Verrocchio, M. C. (2021). MMPI-2 Profile of mothers engaged in parental alienation. *Journal of Family Issues*, *42*, 722–740. https://doi.org/10.1177/0192513X20918393

Roma, P., Marchetti, D., Mazza, C., Ricci, E., Fontanesi, L., & Verrocchio, M. C. (2022). A comparison of MMPI-2 profiles between parental alienation cases and custody cases. *Journal of Child and Family Studies*, *31*, 1196–1206. https://doi.org/10.1007/s10826-021-02076-1

7

THEORIES EXPLAINING PARENTAL ALIENATION

Having explored the behaviours, motivations, and psychological profiles of alienating parents in the preceding chapter, we now turn to the theoretical frameworks that help explain *why* these patterns emerge and *how* they exert such a profound influence on children and family systems. Understanding PA demands more than a description of individual actions; it requires a deep engagement with the relational, systemic, and developmental dynamics that underpin this complex phenomenon.

This chapter introduces and critically examines several major psychological theories that offer explanatory power in the context of PA: attachment theory, family systems theory, psychoanalytic approaches, and Interpersonal Acceptance-Rejection Theory (IPARTheory). Each of these perspectives sheds light on different dimensions of the alienation process: how children internalise distorted relational narratives, how loyalty conflicts are sustained, how unresolved trauma may be transmitted intergenerationally, and how relational bonds are fractured through subtle and coercive means.

These theoretical models also help us move beyond simplistic or pathologising interpretations of alienated families. They provide a language for describing the nuanced psychological and interpersonal mechanisms involved in PA, while also supporting the development of more informed clinical interventions and legal responses. Importantly, these frameworks do not exist in isolation. Rather, they intersect and often reinforce one another, offering an integrated understanding of PA as a form of relational trauma

DOI: 10.4324/9781003630944-10

and, increasingly, as a manifestation of coercive control within the family system.

In tracing these theories, we aim not only to deepen our conceptual grasp of PA but also to highlight their implications for practice, particularly in contexts where alienation is misunderstood, minimised, or contested. By drawing upon these rich and evolving bodies of thought, this chapter lays the groundwork for a more comprehensive, compassionate, and evidence-informed approach to both recognising and responding to parental alienation.

ATTACHMENT THEORY

Parental alienation can be conceptualised fundamentally as an *attachment disorder of the family system*, wherein the child's innate drive to seek proximity, comfort, and security from both caregivers is actively subverted. Rather than forming or maintaining secure connections with both parents, the child is caught in a dynamic that destabilises their sense of relational safety, particularly with the targeted parent, and redirects their attachment needs towards a caregiver who manipulates those needs to serve their own unresolved vulnerabilities.

Bowlby's Attachment Theory

John Bowlby's foundational work on attachment theory emphasises that the early bonds formed between children and their caregivers provide the bedrock for psychological resilience, emotional regulation, and the capacity for healthy relationships throughout life. When these bonds are consistently nurturing, the child develops an internal working model of themselves as worthy of love and others as trustworthy and reliable. However, where attachment is disrupted, particularly through inconsistent, neglectful, or coercive caregiving, the child may develop distorted relational expectations and maladaptive coping strategies.

In cases of parental alienation, attachment theory offers a powerful framework to understand the enactment of alienating behaviours as a defensive response by the alienating parent, whose own attachment system may be compromised. This parent may suffer from unresolved fears of abandonment or betrayal, often rooted in their own developmental trauma. In the post-separation context, such a parent may become excessively dependent on the child for emotional security, effectively co-opting the child's attachment system to meet their own psychological needs.

As a result, the child is drawn into a maladaptive attachment configuration, often marked by emotional enmeshment with the alienating parent. The child's natural need for a bond with both caregivers is gradually eroded as the alienating parent introduces fear, mistrust, or disdain towards the other parent. These tactics, whether overt or covert, actively undermine the child's attachment with the targeted parent, recasting that once secure figure as dangerous, emotionally unavailable, or unworthy of love. Over time, the child internalises these narratives, resulting in a profound rupture in the parent–child bond and the emergence of a false self designed to maintain loyalty to the alienating parent.

This distorted attachment landscape cannot be understood merely as the child's behavioural problem or a function of divorce stress; it reflects a complex interplay of the alienating parent's defensive strategies and the child's desperate attempt to maintain attachment security, even if that means sacrificing a bond with one parent entirely.

The Dynamic-Maturational Model (DMM) of Attachment

The Dynamic-Maturational Model (DMM) of attachment, developed by Dr Patricia Crittenden, extends Bowlby's original framework by considering how attachment strategies evolve in the face of danger, inconsistency, or emotional threat. It focuses on how individuals adapt their attachment behaviour not just to seek safety but also to maximise self-protection in environments where caregivers may be frightening, unreliable, or emotionally overwhelming.

In the context of parental alienation, the DMM allows us to understand the child's attachment behaviours as adaptive responses to a relational environment saturated with coercion and conflicting emotional demands. The alienating parent may present themselves as the sole safe haven, while simultaneously constructing the targeted parent as a source of emotional or physical threat, even where no such threat exists. This creates a double-bind for the child: to remain safe, they must align with the alienating parent and reject the other. The child's attachment system becomes skewed towards strategies that prioritise emotional survival over balanced relational engagement.

The attachment strategies that may emerge in this context include:

- Type A (Compulsive Self-Reliance or Caregiving): The child may suppress their own emotional needs and either become self-sufficient or assume responsibility for the alienating parent's emotional wellbeing. In doing so, the child distances themselves from the targeted parent, who is cast as irrelevant or harmful.
- Type C (Coercive Care-Seeking or Feigned Helplessness): Some children may develop anxious strategies characterised by clinging behaviour, hostility, or exaggerated helplessness – behaviours that ensure continued approval from the alienating parent and maintain alignment against the targeted parent.
- Type A/C (Segregated Systems): In more severe cases, the child may compartmentalise their relational world entirely – displaying warmth and affection only towards the alienating parent, while showing

coldness or fear towards the targeted parent. This split reflects an attempt to resolve conflicting messages by psychologically isolating their internal representations of each parent.

- Loss of Type B (Balanced) Strategies: Ideally, the child would maintain secure relationships with both parents. However, the manipulations inherent in PA actively dismantle this balance, replacing it with defensive strategies that prioritise loyalty over authenticity.

These patterns are not mere behavioural mimicry; they reflect the child's altered attachment system in response to a relational environment distorted by the alienating parent's unmet emotional needs. The alienating parent may project their own fears, mistrust, or unresolved trauma onto the child's relationship with the targeted parent, thus initiating a cycle of misattunement and rejection that the child internalises as truth.

Childress's Attachment-Based Model of Parental Alienation

One of the most distinctive theoretical contributions to the understanding of PA through the lens of attachment theory comes from clinical psychologist Dr Craig Childress, who has developed what he terms the Attachment-Based Model of Parental Alienation (AB-PA). Rather than framing PA as a novel or isolated phenomenon, as earlier models such as Parental Alienation Syndrome (PAS) did, Childress situates it firmly within the established domains of attachment pathology, personality disorder dynamics, and family systems theory.

At the heart of Childress's model is the idea that parental alienation reflects a form of induced attachment trauma, wherein the alienating parent, often described as displaying narcissistic or borderline personality traits (see previous chapter), enacts a pattern of pathogenic parenting. This pattern involves emotional enmeshment, role reversal, and psychological manipulation, whereby the child is subtly coerced into becoming a regulatory object for the alienating parent's own unresolved attachment anxieties. In essence, the child is co-opted into the parent's internal world, and asked to carry the emotional burden of the parent's historical trauma.

Childress outlines three diagnostic indicators that signal the presence of this form of induced relational disturbance in the child:

1. Suppression of the attachment system: The child exhibits an anomalous and rigid severance of attachment to the targeted parent, not due to maltreatment but through psychological coercion.
2. Narcissistic/borderline-like traits: The child displays grandiosity, entitlement, and a lack of empathy towards the rejected parent – traits that reflect an internalised replication of the alienating parent's relational style.
3. Delusional or fixed false beliefs: The child forms rigid, factually ungrounded negative beliefs about the targeted parent, resistant to evidence and contrary to the child's own prior relationship history.

These features, according to Childress, are not coincidental. They emerge from the systematic suppression of the child's authentic attachment system and its replacement with a distorted relational schema aligned with the alienating parent. The result is not merely alienation but a reconfiguration of the child's psychological architecture, built upon defensive, maladaptive attachment responses.

Childress also emphasises causality. He argues that the behaviours observed in the alienated child are not spontaneous or idiosyncratic but *induced*, a result of psychological processes initiated by the alienating parent, whose own unresolved attachment trauma is projected onto the child. This process constitutes what Childress calls a trauma reenactment narrative, in which the child is enlisted into replaying the alienating parent's emotional history. The alienated parent is recast in the role of the original attachment figure who once failed or abandoned the alienating parent, thereby justifying the child's rejection within the distorted emotional logic of the alienating system.

In terms of treatment, Childress proposes a structured intervention strategy based on protective separation: a time-limited, therapeutically supported removal of the child from the influence of the alienating parent. During this period, the child is given a safe psychological space in which to reconnect with the targeted parent and begin to restore their suppressed attachment system. Therapeutic work in this context does not focus on blame or adjudication but on restoring the child's capacity for authentic emotional experience and relational reciprocity. Once the attachment bond shows signs of reactivation, structured re-engagement with the alienating parent can be cautiously reintroduced.

What distinguishes Childress's model is not only its theoretical grounding in attachment and personality theory but its rejection of PAS as a freestanding syndrome. Instead, he advocates for integration within existing psychological frameworks, including DSM-recognised constructs such as *Child Psychological Abuse (V995.51)*. In doing so, he seeks to reposition PA not as a controversial or fringe concept but as a specific manifestation of well-documented relational trauma.

While Childress's work has been the subject of both interest and critique, particularly in its prescriptive diagnostic structure and emphasis on pathologising the alienating parent, it offers a compelling synthesis of clinical theory and practice. Most importantly, it reinforces the idea that at the core of parental alienation lies a profound rupture in the attachment system, one that is neither spontaneous nor benign, but actively constructed through the dynamics of unresolved parental trauma, misdirected emotional regulation, and systemic failure to intervene.

Attachment Approaches: Summary

The deliberate erosion of a child's attachment to a once trusted parent constitutes a profound psychological injury. It not only deprives the child of emotional security in the present but also distorts their internal working models of self and others; models that shape future relationships, self-worth, and the capacity to regulate emotions. When a child is coerced into rejecting a safe and loving parent, their developmental trajectory is redirected through a lens of mistrust, fear, and emotional confusion. This disorganisation at the heart of the attachment system can have enduring effects, often manifesting in anxiety, relational instability, and identity disturbance well into adulthood.

Given the seriousness of these consequences, clinicians must attune to the attachment dynamics at play. Understanding the dual process, wherein the alienating parent exploits the child to manage their own attachment insecurities, and the child adopts maladaptive strategies to maintain psychological coherence, enables more precise and compassionate intervention. Effective therapeutic work must support the child in reconstructing a coherent and secure representation of the rejected parent, while also addressing the relational dysfunction that underpins the alienation. This requires not only clinical sensitivity but also systemic thinking, as any attempt to restore attachment bonds must contend with the powerful psychological and emotional structures that have come to define the child's relational world.

PSYCHOANALYTIC APPROACHES

While attachment theory frames parental alienation as a disruption in the child's capacity to form secure bonds, psychoanalytic approaches dig deeper into the intrapsychic dynamics underlying such disruptions. These approaches, particularly those drawing from object relations theory, offer insights into how alienation emerges not only from interpersonal conflict but also from unresolved psychological trauma, transgenerational patterns, and defensive processes that become embedded in the child's developing sense of self.

Object Relations and the Concept of Splitting

Object relations theory posits that a child's early experiences with caregivers are internalised to form enduring "objects"; mental representations of self, other, and relationship. These internalised objects are not just memories but also active psychological structures that shape how the child interprets future relationships. Healthy development requires the integration of positive and negative experiences into a cohesive sense of others as both loving and frustrating, dependable and fallible.

However, when emotional environments are unstable, overwhelming, or coercively misattuned, the child may resort to splitting as a primitive defence. Splitting is a process through which the child maintains a sense of emotional safety by dividing relational experiences into binary categories: "good" and "bad," "safe" and "dangerous." In the context of parental alienation, this manifests as idealisation of the aligned parent and total devaluation of the targeted parent, a pattern that is developmentally regressive and psychologically protective in the short term but harmful in the long run.

The splitting seen in alienated children is not simply a behavioural rejection of one parent; it is a deeply embedded psychological mechanism that enables the child to manage unbearable conflict and loyalty binds. It also reflects the child's alignment with the psychological defences of the alienating parent, who may themselves be operating from a split internal world. Over time, this dynamic consolidates into a rigid internal structure that prevents emotional integration, trust, and relational ambivalence, hallmarks of healthy psychological maturity.

THE WORK OF KAREN AND NICK WOODALL

Karen and Nick Woodall have been among the most influential practitioners working at the intersection of psychoanalytic theory, child development, and family law in the context of parental alienation. Through their clinical work at the Family Separation Clinic (established in the UK in 2010), they have developed a multi-layered conceptual and therapeutic model that combines psychoanalytic insight with practical intervention strategies, particularly for use in high-conflict custody cases.

Their core conceptualisation of parental alienation frames it not simply as a contact refusal but as a pathological alignment of the child with one parent, to the exclusion and rejection of the other. Crucially, they view the child's overt rejection as a *symptom* rather than a root cause. It is the outcome of sustained psychological processes involving coercive control, role confusion, and emotional triangulation, rather than the result of the rejected parent's conduct per se.

At the heart of their psychoanalytic framing is the concept of splitting (as described above). The alienated child, in the grip of primitive defences, experiences one parent (usually the aligned) as entirely safe and good, and the other (usually the rejected) as wholly unsafe or bad. The capacity to hold mixed feelings, what psychoanalytic theorists call ambivalence, is lost. This defence enables the child to manage intolerable anxiety, especially when the aligned parent has conveyed either overt or subtle messages that love for the other parent is disloyal or dangerous.

The Woodalls also describe the child's psychological state in terms of self-alienation. The child becomes estranged not only from one parent but also from their own prior experiences, memories, and emotional truth. In this sense, PA is not simply a rupture in the external relationship; it is a fracturing of the internal relational world, and a loss of access to parts of the self associated with the targeted parent.

Several key mechanisms structure the Woodalls' psychoanalytic and clinical understanding of PA:

- The Transition Bridge: The Woodalls propose that children require a psychological "bridge" to move between households after separation. Where this bridge is absent or undermined, due to fear, boundary violations, or unresolved inter-parental hostility, the child may experience transitions as psychologically unsafe, reinforcing rigid alignment with one parent and rejection of the other.
- Power, Control, and Emotional Enmeshment: In many cases, the aligned parent exerts emotional control over the child, often driven by their own unresolved fears of abandonment or betrayal. The child's dependency and fear are leveraged, consciously or unconsciously, to maintain an exclusive bond, in which the child is not permitted psychological independence or loyalty to both parents.
- Transgenerational Trauma and Repetition: The Woodalls highlight the transgenerational nature of alienation, observing that patterns of estrangement, boundary violation, and unresolved trauma often repeat across generations. In this view, the alienating parent may be re-enacting their own childhood experience of loss or rejection, projecting unresolved trauma into the current relationship through the child.

Clinical Application: Assessment, Intervention, and Recovery

The Woodalls' work has had significant practical impact in both therapeutic and forensic settings. Their clinical protocols include:

- Differentiation of Cases: They distinguish between *pure alienation*, *hybrid cases* (involving elements of justified rejection), and *justified estrangement*, stressing the importance of accurate assessment before intervention. Misidentification, they argue, risks exacerbating harm.
- Treatment Pathways: In severe cases, they advocate for residence transfer, a carefully managed change of primary residence from the aligned to the rejected parent. This is framed not as a punitive measure but as a therapeutic necessity to break the coercive dynamic and allow the child's authentic attachment system to re-emerge.
- Post-Transfer Therapeutic Work: Crucially, they emphasise that the work does not end with residence change. Ongoing therapeutic intervention is required to help the child re-integrate fragmented experiences, re-establish ambivalence, and recover a sense of coherent identity. This involves careful testing of resilience and adaptation in the child's re-engagement with the previously rejected parent.
- Early Intervention: They advocate for early recognition and response before alienation becomes entrenched, stressing that mild cases can escalate rapidly without timely support.

Their 2017 book, *Understanding Parental Alienation: Learning to Cope, Helping to Heal*, articulates their model in both clinical and legal terms, offering a bridge between psychoanalytic understanding and actionable frameworks for professionals.

The Woodalls' work makes clear that reversing parental alienation is not a matter of restoring contact alone; it is a matter of psychological integration. The alienated child is not merely misinformed; they are in psychological conflict, using primitive defences to preserve a sense of safety in an emotionally coercive environment. Effective intervention must therefore move beyond behaviour management or legal adjudication. It must create the conditions in which the child can again tolerate relational complexity, recover access to their own emotional truth, and re-integrate previously disowned aspects of both the self and the rejected parent.

In this sense, psychoanalytic approaches do not just describe what alienation is; they illuminate why it is so damaging, how it becomes entrenched, and what must occur for genuine healing to begin.

FAMILY SYSTEMS THEORY

Family systems theory, most notably developed by Murray Bowen, offers a valuable framework for understanding PA as not merely an individual pathology but a systemic dysfunction embedded within the relational patterns of the family unit. At its core, the theory posits that family members operate as an emotional system, interdependent, reciprocal, and patterned across generations, such that the behaviour of one member cannot be fully understood without considering its impact on, and connection to, others.

From this perspective, PA is not simply a matter of a child rejecting a parent but a symptom of deeper, systemic disturbances, particularly those activated during periods of acute family stress, such as high-conflict separation or divorce. The rejection of a previously loved parent by a child is thus viewed not as an isolated choice or purely psychological reaction but as the visible outcome of dysfunctional relational patterns that involve all members of the family system, especially those dynamics that operate below the level of conscious awareness.

Triangulation and Coalition Formation

A central concept in family systems theory is triangulation: a dynamic in which two family members form a coalition against a third in order to reduce anxiety or maintain relational equilibrium. In the context of PA, this often manifests as a coalition between the alienating parent and the child, who become psychologically aligned against the targeted parent. This triadic configuration serves to stabilise the alienating parent's emotional position, often rooted in unresolved anger, fear of abandonment, or loss of control, but does so at the cost of the child's independent emotional development and secure attachment to both parents.

Rather than being encouraged to maintain differentiated relationships with each parent, the child is drawn into an inappropriate loyalty bind, in which rejecting the targeted parent is presented, either explicitly or implicitly, as a necessary condition for preserving closeness with the alienating parent. In such scenarios, the child is not acting autonomously but is functioning as an extension of the alienating parent's emotional system, participating in a relational script that prioritises the needs of the parent over the child's psychological integrity.

Boundary Distortions and Role Reversal

Another key tenet of family systems theory is the importance of maintaining clear generational boundaries between parents and children. In alienating family systems, these boundaries are frequently violated. The alienating parent may enmesh the child into adult concerns, burdening them with emotional responsibilities that exceed their developmental capacity. This can include confiding in the child about legal disputes, encouraging the child to monitor or critique the other parent, or relying on the child for emotional validation and companionship in ways that invert the expected caregiver–child dynamic.

Such boundary violations result in role corruption, where the child assumes a protective, or even spousal, role towards the alienating parent. In order to fulfil this role and maintain harmony within the dyadic alliance, the child may suppress their own attachment needs and adopt the alienating parent's narrative as their own, eventually leading to overt rejection of the targeted parent. Importantly, these dynamics are not always the result of conscious manipulation; they can arise from deeply entrenched systemic patterns, often spanning multiple generations.

Intergenerational Transmission and Systemic Repetition

Family systems theory also accounts for the transgenerational transmission of dysfunctional patterns. In many cases, the alienating parent may themselves be enacting unresolved relational trauma from their own family of origin, such as prior experiences of rejection, neglect, or unresolved conflict with a parental figure. These unresolved dynamics are then reactivated in the current family system, particularly under the stress of separation or loss, and re-enacted through the child's relationship with the targeted parent. In this sense, PA can be understood as a repetition of unprocessed emotional material, projected into the next generation.

Implications for Intervention

Viewing PA through the lens of family systems theory shifts the focus from individual pathology to relational patterns and systemic imbalance.

Interventions informed by this perspective must therefore go beyond individual therapy or custody arrangements to address the entire family structure, with particular attention to:

- Identifying and disrupting triangulated alliances;
- Restoring appropriate generational boundaries;
- Supporting emotional differentiation in the child;
- Addressing unresolved trauma or dysfunction in the parental subsystem.

Such interventions may include systemic family therapy, psychoeducation, or, in severe cases, restructuring the family environment (e.g., residence transfer) to create the conditions necessary for the child to develop healthy, autonomous relationships with both parents. Crucially, this model reinforces that the child's rejection is not the problem in itself; it is a signal of deeper systemic distress that must be resolved at the level of family functioning.

INTERPERSONAL ACCEPTANCE-REJECTION THEORY AND THE CONSEQUENCES OF PARENTAL ALIENATION

At its psychological core, PA represents an experience of perceived parental rejection, a child's belief that one parent is no longer loving, supportive, or emotionally available. This rejection may be factitious, induced by another adult, or reinforced through systemic dynamics, but the developmental and emotional experience for the child is real and consequential. Interpersonal Acceptance-Rejection Theory (IPARTheory) is a global, evidence-based framework that examines how perceived acceptance or rejection by significant others, especially parents, influences psychological adjustment. Originating in the work of Ronald P. Rohner, IPARTheory offers a powerful complement to attachment theory and family systems approaches by emphasising subjective perception and cultural generalisability. In the context of PA, IPARTheory helps illuminate why the emotional consequences of alienation are often profound, enduring, and psychologically corrosive.

Core Concepts in IPARTheory

At the heart of IPARTheory is the assertion that humans have an innate, biologically based need for emotional acceptance from those to whom they are emotionally attached, particularly parents. When children perceive themselves to be accepted, characterised by warmth, affection, and support, they are more likely to develop secure, resilient, and socially competent personalities. Conversely, perceived rejection, marked by coldness, hostility, neglect, or indifference, is consistently associated with a range of adverse outcomes, including anxiety, depression, aggression, low self-esteem, and impaired emotional regulation.

IPARTheory is organised around three interrelated sub-theories:

- Personality Subtheory: Identifies consistent patterns in personality development linked to experiences of perceived acceptance or rejection.
- Coping Subtheory: Explores why some individuals are more resilient to perceived rejection than others, incorporating temperament, cultural expectations, and relational supports.
- Sociocultural Systems Subtheory: Examines how the experience and consequences of rejection vary – or remain consistent – across diverse cultural settings.

Crucially, research across more than 60 nations and cultures has found remarkable universality in the developmental consequences of parental rejection, making IPARTheory one of the most cross-culturally validated frameworks in developmental psychology (Rohner, 2021).

Parental Alienation as Perceived Rejection

Within this framework, parental alienation can be understood as an experience of induced or manipulated rejection. The child is led to believe that one parent is fundamentally unloving, unsafe, or emotionally unavailable, often through the coercive influence of the other parent. This rejection may be based on exaggerated or fabricated narratives, but its psychological impact is consistent with the core predictions of IPARTheory.

Even in the absence of objective harm, the subjective experience of rejection, whether constructed or real, activates the same psychological vulnerabilities: chronic emotional insecurity, relational mistrust, diminished self-worth, and difficulties forming stable attachments later in life. The alienated child not only loses a meaningful relationship with one parent but also internalises a set of cognitive and emotional schemas associated with parental non-acceptance.

Furthermore, the alienating parent's behaviour may also contribute to feelings of rejection, albeit masked as alignment or loyalty. When a child is enlisted in an adult's emotional agenda, expected to sever ties with a loving parent, and discouraged from expressing ambivalence or autonomy, they may experience subtle but significant violations of emotional safety and acceptance from both parents, further compounding the psychological risk.

Long-Term Outcomes: "As You Sow, So Shall You Reap"

IPARTheory also highlights the lifespan consequences of perceived rejection. Research shows that adults who felt rejected by their parents in childhood often exhibit reduced empathy, diminished caregiving motivation, and, in many cases, counter-rejection towards their now elderly or dependent parents. In Rohner and Ali's (2025) *Global Perspectives*, this phenomenon is captured by the aphorism: *"As you sow, so shall you reap."*

In the context of PA, this means that the alienating parent, while temporarily securing a child's alliance, may ultimately undermine their own future relationship with that child. If the child later comes to recognise the manipulation or loses trust in the parent who induced the alienation, a reversal of emotional allegiance may occur. Such cycles can have profound implications not only for individual development but also for intergenerational family functioning.

Implications for Assessment and Intervention

IPARTheory offers several critical insights for practitioners working with alienated children and their families:

- Assessment should prioritise the child's perceived emotional experience, not merely behavioural compliance or reported histories. This includes exploring whether the child feels loved, safe, and emotionally supported by both parents.
- Rejection narratives must be interrogated carefully, especially when they appear rehearsed, exaggerated, or unsupported by objective evidence. Interventions should work to deconstruct these beliefs and re-establish more realistic relational appraisals.
- Cultural sensitivity is essential (more on this in Chapter 8). IPARTheory's sociocultural systems model can guide clinicians in adapting approaches to different familial and community contexts, recognising how norms around obedience, loyalty, and parental authority shape children's experiences.
- Prevention is possible. If PA is conceptualised as a form of psychological rejection, then early efforts to preserve acceptance, warmth, and open communication across both parental relationships may reduce the risk of alignment and rejection dynamics becoming entrenched.

IPARTheory deepens our understanding of the psychological cost of parental alienation by framing it as an experience of interpersonal rejection, with cross-culturally validated consequences for mental health, relational capacity, and developmental trajectory. It invites us to move beyond legal and behavioural definitions of alienation and focus on the child's internal experience; how they make meaning of parental behaviour, and how those meanings shape who they become.

In doing so, it reinforces the urgency of early, emotionally attuned, and culturally informed interventions; not simply to restore contact, but to rebuild the child's sense of being unconditionally accepted and loved by both parents. Only then can the developmental damage of alienation begin to heal.

INTEGRATING THEORETICAL PERSPECTIVES: WHY PARENTAL ALIENATION HAPPENS AND WHAT IT DOES

At the most basic level, attachment theory explains that children have a fundamental need for security, comfort, and emotional attunement from their primary caregivers. When parents separate, the child's attachment system becomes activated by threat and uncertainty. In high-conflict contexts, one parent may exploit this vulnerability by enmeshing the child in a maladaptive alignment, offering pseudo-security while undermining the child's relationship with the other parent. The child, in turn, may suppress their need for the rejected parent to maintain emotional harmony with the aligned one, distorting their internal working models of love, safety, and trust.

Psychoanalytic theory, particularly object relations, deepens this account by revealing how alienation is sustained through primitive psychological defences. The aligned parent may operate from unresolved trauma, projecting their own fears of abandonment or betrayal onto the child's relationship with the other parent. The child, drawn into this emotional economy, adopts splitting, dividing their relational world into "all good" and "all bad," to preserve psychological coherence. This binary logic is protective in the short term but leaves the child unable to integrate mixed feelings or tolerate relational complexity.

Family systems theory provides the structural map for these dynamics. It explains how triangulation, coalitions, and boundary violations escalate during familial crisis. The child is often recruited into a loyalty bind, where rejecting one parent becomes a condition of closeness with the other. Generational roles become blurred, emotional responsibilities are inverted, and the child's psychological independence is subverted to maintain system "stability." PA, from this view, is not merely a parenting issue; it is a symptom of a dysfunctional family system struggling to manage anxiety, loss, and unresolved conflict.

Finally, IPARTheory reframes the child's experience in terms of perceived parental rejection. Whether the rejection is based on actual neglect or is artificially induced by the aligned parent, the child internalises it as real. The psychological result, consistent across cultures, is a cascade of adverse outcomes: diminished self-worth, relational distrust, behavioural dysregulation, and long-term emotional vulnerability. IPARTheory captures the subjective reality of the child, emphasising that harm occurs not only when a parent is absent but also when they are emotionally discredited in the child's eyes.

What Parental Alienation Does: Psychological and Developmental Impact

Together, these theories describe a process that begins in the family system, takes root in the child's attachment dynamics, is maintained by unconscious defence mechanisms, and is experienced as interpersonal rejection. The consequences are layered and enduring:

- Attachment disturbance: The child loses a secure bond with a previously trusted caregiver and may form anxious or disorganised attachments moving forward.
- Distorted internal representations: The alienated parent is seen as wholly bad or dangerous, while the aligned parent is idealised. The child loses access to authentic memories and balanced emotional experiences.
- Role corruption and identity confusion: Children may become parentified, emotionally burdened, or disconnected from age-appropriate developmental tasks.
- Emotional dysregulation and self-alienation: In attempting to maintain harmony with the aligned parent, the child suppresses their own emotional truth – leading to shame, confusion, and long-term difficulties in emotional expression.
- Relational consequences across the lifespan: As IPARTheory shows, children who feel rejected by a parent are at greater risk for depression, aggression, and mistrust in adult relationships. They may also come to reject the aligned parent later in life, perpetuating intergenerational cycles of estrangement.

An Integrated Model for Conceptualising PA

What emerges from this integration is a multi-level explanatory model:

Level	*Core Concept*	*Key Mechanism*
Attachment	Disrupted emotional security	Child withdraws from targeted parent to maintain stability
Psychoanalytic	Unconscious defences and projections	Splitting, projection, identification with aggressor
Family Systems	Systemic instability and triangulation	Enmeshment, role reversal, loyalty conflicts
IPARTheory	Subjective experience of rejection	Internalised belief of being unloved or unwanted

This model (See Figure 7.1) allows professionals, clinicians, legal experts, social workers, and educators to see PA not as a single event or behavioural issue but as a complex psychological and relational syndrome. It is best addressed not by blame or simplistic solutions but by interventions that are developmentally attuned, systemically informed, and emotionally integrative.

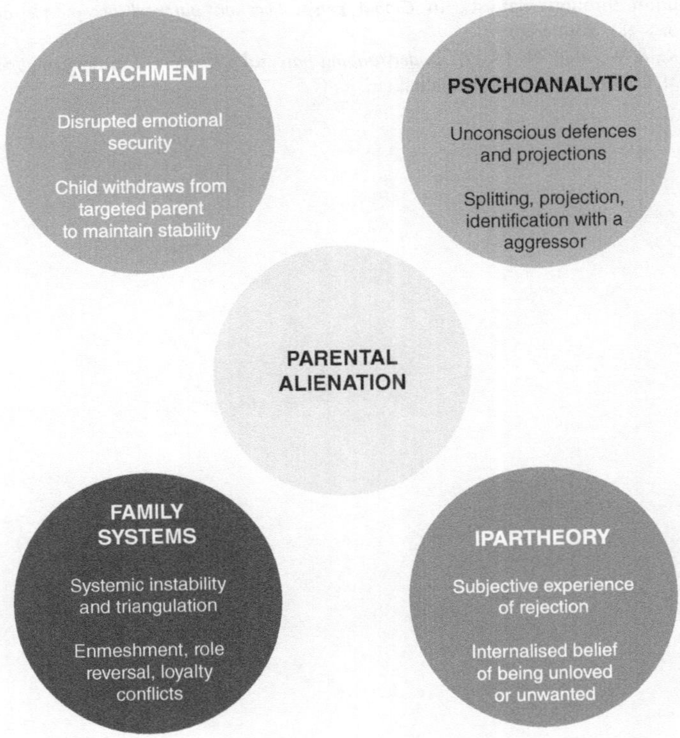

Figure 7.1 Theoretical frameworks proposed to explain parental alienation.

BIBLIOGRAPHY

Childress, C. (2015). *An Attachment-Based Model of Parental Alienation*. Oaksong Press.

Crittenden, P. M., Landini, A., Speiker, S. J., & Grey, B. (2021). Using parental attachment in family court proceedings: DMM theory about the adult attachment interview. *Child Abuse Review*. https://doi.org/10.1002/car.2730

Keller, M. N., & Noone, R. J. (Eds.). (2019). *Handbook of Bowen family systems theory and research methods: A systems model for family research*. Routledge.

Lowenstein, L. F. (2010). Attachment theory and parental alienation. *Journal of Divorce and Remarriage*, 51, 157–168. https://doi.org/10.1080/10502551003597808

Ripoll-Núñez, K., & Carrillo, S. (2016). Adult intimate relationships: Linkages between interpersonal acceptance-rejection theory and adult attachment theory. *Online Readings in Psychology and Culture*, 6(2). https://doi.org/10.9707/2307-0919.1149

Rohner, R. P. (2021). Introduction to interpersonal acceptance-rejection theory (IPARTheory) and evidence. *Online Readings in Psychology and Culture*, 6(1). https://doi.org/10.9707/2307-0919.1055

Rohner, R. P., & Ali, S. (2025). Interpersonal acceptance-rejection theory (IPARTheory): From conception through maturity. In *Global perspectives on parental acceptance and rejection* (pp. 3–38). Routledge.

Woodall, K., & Woodall, N. (2017). *Understanding parental alienation: Learning to cope, helping to heal*. Charles C Thomas Publisher, Ltd.

8

CULTURE, CONTEXT, AND THE CONDITIONS THAT SUSTAIN PARENTAL ALIENATION

Parental alienation does not occur in a vacuum. While much of the clinical and theoretical literature rightly focuses on individual psychology and family dynamics, these are always embedded within broader social and cultural ecosystems. Legal systems, gender norms, professional ideologies, and even the language we use to describe parenting and family breakdown all influence how parental alienation is expressed, understood, and responded to. In this chapter, we shift our focus to examine the structural and societal conditions that enable alienation to take root and, too often, to go unchallenged. Drawing on ecological systems theory, psychosocial theory, and cultural psychology, this chapter explores how power, identity, and ideology intersect with personal trauma to shape the lived realities of alienated families. In doing so, we aim to illuminate the socio-cultural scaffolding of parental alienation and challenge the myth that it is solely a private family matter.

APPLYING THE ECOLOGICAL MODEL TO PARENTAL ALIENATION

In the preceding chapter(s), we focused largely on the individual (child, alienating parent, targeted parent) and the immediate relational microsystem (family, parent–child interactions). Bronfenbrenner's ecological model (See Figure 8.1) reminds us that these dynamics are embedded within broader

DOI: 10.4324/9781003630944-11

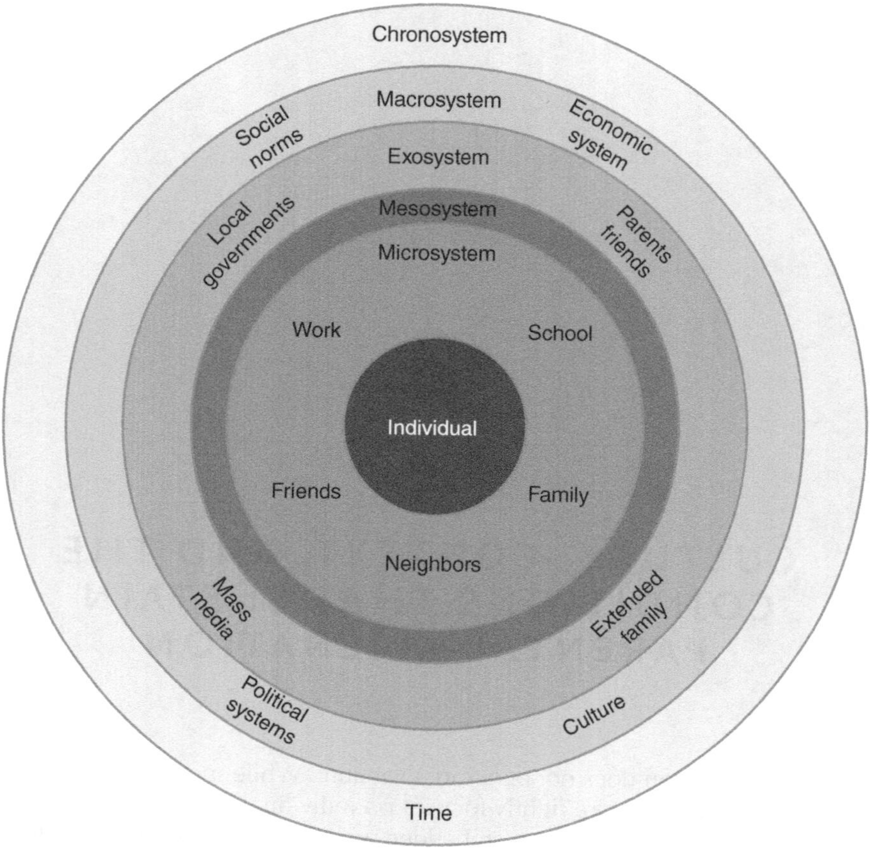

Figure 8.1 Bronfenbrenner's ecological model.

systems that shape possibilities for behaviour, resistance, and remediation. When we extend our lens to the mesosystem, exosystem, macrosystem, and chronosystem, we can better understand why PA arises, why it persists, and what levers of change might exist beyond the individual or dyadic level.

Crucially, as Dr Stan Korosi advocates, we must not treat PA purely as a private disorder. Rather, we should embed it in social, structural, and policy contexts, exploring how legal regimes, discourses of power, institutional norms, and public health systems intersect with psychological processes. Incorporating structural and social analysis helps us integrate paradigms of formulation, assessment, remediation, and socio-legal response in a more holistic and realistic way.

Below, I map how each ecological level might contribute to the onset, amplification, or mitigation of parental alienation, and highlight intersections with your prior theoretical models.

The Mesosystem: Interconnections Between Microsystems

The mesosystem encompasses the connections between two or more microsystems in which the child is embedded, such as the relationships between family and school, between therapeutic or legal systems and the home environment, or between peer groups and parental networks. In the context of PA, the mesosystem is especially important because it is where spillover effects and cross-system influences occur.

How the mesosystem may influence or exacerbate PA:

- Legal–Family interface: Family courts, mediators, custody evaluators, child protection agencies, mental health professionals, and domestic violence services all represent microsystems that intersect with the family. Their practices, biases, and decisions feed back into the home. For example, court delays, misinterpretation of alienation, or adversarial custody processes can intensify conflict and drive deeper alienation.
- School, peers, community as carriers of narrative: In high-conflict separations, the alienating parent may attempt to mobilise school staff, teachers, counsellors, or classmates to validate the child's negative views of the targeted parent. This gives additional social legitimacy to the alienating discourse, magnifying the child's internal conflict and isolating the rejected parent further.
- Therapeutic or professional networks: Where the alienating parent finds sympathetic therapists, coaches, or legal advocates, these alliances may reinforce alienation narratives and inhibit corrective feedback. Conversely, if the targeted parent has stronger alliances in the therapeutic/educational community, they may gain support for reunification efforts.
- Extended family, social supports, and religious institutions: These may function as bridging microsystems. For example, if grandparents, aunts/uncles, or community mentors maintain contact with the targeted parent and oppose the alienating narrative, they can buffer against total relational collapse. Alternatively, if extended family supports the alienating discourse, they contribute to systemic isolation.

In effect, the mesosystem is where external systems and family life collide, and where PA may either be reinforced or intercepted.

The Exosystem: Indirect Influences and Institutional Contexts

The exosystem refers to environments that do not directly involve the child but nonetheless influence their world through their effects on the parents or family system. In PA, the exosystem is particularly potent because many driving forces operate at the institutional or structural level.

Key exosystem factors relevant to PA:

- Legal and judicial systems: Legal statutes, court precedents, family violence laws, and case-processing norms (e.g., how allegations are handled, timelines, and evidentiary standards) exert a strong influence over what kinds of parenting or alienating behaviour go unchecked or are punished. Korosi argues that many jurisdictions still default to gendered frameworks or presume shared care without adequate safeguards, thereby inadvertently enabling alienation.
- Child protection and social services: The practices of social services – how they classify parental alienation (or whether they classify it at all), whether they intervene, and whether they treat it as a form of emotional abuse – make a difference in how families are held accountable or allowed to continue destructive dynamics. If social services treat PA superficially or not at all, alienating behaviours may escalate unchecked.
- Mental health and clinical norms: The standards for diagnosis, insurance coverage, availability of specialist therapists, and professional training influence what kinds of interventions are possible. If clinicians lack access or training to treat alienation meaningfully, families may default to adversarial legal routes.
- Media, public narratives, and professional discourse: The public, legal, and professional discourses around divorce, "bad parents," and children's "choice" shape how alienation is understood (or denied). The exosystem includes the legal, journalistic, academic, and policy discourses that either normalise or pathologise PA or turn it into a political issue. Korosi emphasises that alienating discourse is not merely interpersonal; it is discursive violence, normalising defamation and vilification within relational systems.
- Welfare, economic systems, employment, and social inequality: The economic stressors on parents (e.g., job insecurity, economic disparity, housing, and access to legal representation) can strain parental capacity, fuel resentment, or limit the ability to maintain contact. Social policies (child support, custody presumption, and legal aid) may implicitly favour one parent over another or trivialise relational harms.

Thus, even though the child may not directly engage with exosystem actors, those actors shape the structural possibilities and constraints under which alienation actions occur.

The Macrosystem: Culture, Ideology, and Discourse

The macrosystem encompasses overarching cultural values, ideologies, symbolic systems, laws, norms, and belief structures. It is here that we locate the structural and discursive scaffolding within which PA is either legitimised or resisted.

Macrosystem dynamics relevant to parental alienation:

- Cultural models of parenting, divorce and custody: In cultures that emphasise maternal primacy, sole custody, or patriarchal assumptions about family roles, the non-residential parent is culturally marginalised even before alienation begins. These cultural scripts may tacitly support alienating behaviour by pathologising efforts to maintain contact.
- Discursive violence and narrative power: Korosi speaks of *alienating discourse*, the narratives, symbols, and linguistic practices that recast the targeted parent as villainous, the child as a loyal victim, and the alienating parent as the protector. These narratives mirror broader societal discourses about family, identity, gender, and power.
- Ideologies of individualism, autonomy, and choice: In highly individualistic cultures, the idea that a child might "choose" a parent or reject contact may be more socially acceptable or less questioned. The rhetoric of personal autonomy may be weaponised to mask coercion; "The child's choice" becomes a legitimising trope.
- Legal-political frameworks and gendered norms: Macrosystem forces include how law, public policy, and political ideologies conceive of family, children's rights, and parental authority. For example, if family law treats alienation as a custody dispute rather than relational harm, the systemic response may be inadequate. Korosi criticises the "gendered paradigm" in many jurisdictions that frames family violence through a lens of male violence towards women, often neglecting how alienation operates across gender lines.
- Structural inequality, stigma, and marginalisation: Race, class, gender, mobility status, and social capital all influence which families are more vulnerable to alienation and less able to mobilise resources. The macrosystem shapes which voices are legitimised or silenced in public and legal arenas.

The macrosystem, then, is the ideological soil in which alienation discourse grows. It sets the terms for what is considered acceptable, credible, or dismissible.

The Chronosystem: Time, Transitions, and Change

Finally, the chronosystem adds the dimension of time; it examines how changes across time (life events, generational shifts, legal reforms, and cultural evolution) influence the risk and trajectory of PA.

Chronosystem considerations in PA:

- Life transitions and tipping points: Divorce, remarriage, relocation, legal rulings, adolescence, and loss can serve as inflection points when latent tensions in loyalty, identity, or control surface into overt alienation.

- Historical shifts in family law, policy, and ideology: Over decades, societal beliefs about custody, gender roles, and child autonomy evolve. For instance, a shift towards shared parenting presumptions, or increased recognition of emotional abuse, may alter how PA is framed and influence legal outcomes.
- Generational transmission: Patterns of relational alienation, unresolved trauma, boundary dysfunction, or parent–child estrangement may be passed down across generations. The chronosystem captures how past family history shapes present vulnerability to alienation.
- Cultural change and discursive shifts: Over time, public awareness campaigns, media portrayals, judicial precedents, and scholarly work may shift how PA is understood and managed. These temporal evolutions influence both risk and remedy.
- Evolving theoretical frameworks: Early models of PA, particularly those centred on individual pathology or controversial constructs such as Parental Alienation Syndrome (PAS), have shaped both public scepticism and professional hesitancy. However, the theoretical shift towards relational, systemic, and trauma-informed understandings represents a positive development within the chronosystem, demonstrating how conceptual evolution over time can refine both assessment and intervention approaches.

INTEGRATING ECOLOGICAL LEVELS WITH PRIOR THEORIES AND KOROSI'S STRUCTURAL CALL

By overlaying the ecological model on top of your existing theoretical integration (attachment, psychoanalytic, systems, IPARTheory), you create a multi-tiered framework that links individual psychology, relational patterns, and broader sociocultural forces.

- The microsystem remains the ground of direct interaction – where attachment is built or undermined, and where splitting or relational defences play out.
- The mesosystem is the zone where external systems (courts, schools, therapy, and community) either reinforce or disrupt alienation narratives.
- The exosystem encompasses institutional levers – legal systems, social services, and discursive networks – that shape the boundary conditions for what behaviour is permitted or obscured.
- The macrosystem grounds the ideological, normative, and discursive frameworks that make alienation intelligible or invisible.
- The chronosystem reminds us that these patterns evolve, mutate, or reverse over time.

Korosi's call for social and structural formulations finds its natural home in this layered model. He insists that PA cannot be reduced to psychopathology or dyadic conflict but must be understood as a discursive, structural, and relational harm, a problem not only of families but also of society.

In practice, then, intervention should not stop at the child–parent dyad. Effective strategies might include:

- Reforming legal and custody systems to recognise emotional abuse or alienation as harm.
- Training professionals (judges, social workers, therapists) to detect alienating discourse and resist its legitimation.
- Creating community supports, peer networks, and public awareness to counter narratives of alienation.
- Monitoring cultural scripts (media, policy, public rhetoric) that normalise "parental estrangement."
- Ensuring longitudinal monitoring of high-conflict families to detect escalation or shift over time.

MACROSYSTEM AND CULTURAL VARIATION IN PARENTAL ALIENATION

So, the macrosystem in Bronfenbrenner's model encompasses the broad cultural, ideological, legal, and discursive structures within which families operate. In the case of PA, the macrosystem does more than provide context; it actively *constitutes* how PA is understood, contested, legitimised, or suppressed. The very way scholars and practitioners conceptualise intersecting cultural stereotypes, legal traditions, gender norms, and public discourse about separation and parenthood shapes PA. What counts as "alienation" in one society may be dismissed, pathologised, or silenced in another.

Below, I outline how different national contexts reflect differing stages or orientations of PA discourse, and how these are inextricably tied to the macrosystem's cultural beliefs and structural assumptions.

The United States and Canada: Litigation, Expert Witnessing, and Polarised Discourse

In the US and Canada, PA discourse tends to be litigation-driven and deeply entwined with adversarial custody battles. The courts, mental health experts, and advocacy groups play a strong role in shaping the macro narrative around PA. The legacy of Richard Gardner's Parental Alienation Syndrome (PAS) remains influential in many legal circles, even as many clinicians and feminist scholars criticise it as oversimplified or abusive.

Here, the macrosystem supports the notion of individual liability and pathology. Alienation is also often framed as a "defence" or technical manoeuvre in custody litigation, rather than as a relational or structural phenomenon. Such framing tends to discount broader socio-cultural or structural forces, such as gender bias, power differentials, or institutional failure. Critics argue that, in courts without deep literacy in domestic violence, PA is sometimes misused to dismiss genuine claims of abuse.

The United Kingdom and Australia: Institutional Shielding, Professional Caution, and Evolving Recognition

In the UK and Australia, PA discourse tends to be mediated by professional gatekeepers: family courts, children's guardians, social services, and psychological associations. The macrosystem in these contexts often emphasises child protection, domestic violence frameworks, and safeguarding, which sometimes clash or compete with PA narratives.

In the UK, courts have been wary of PA, citing insufficient empirical support. The notion of PA tends to be used more cautiously, often under the heading of relational alienation or parenting interference, and is sometimes subsumed under emotional abuse or neglect categories. The institutional frameworks here shape a more conservative reception: PA must be substantiated carefully so as not to override other protective imperatives.

In Australia, too, discourse around PA is growing, but it is often modulated by robust legislative frameworks for domestic violence and child protection. These macro structures make courts, social services, and therapists more alert to misuse of power and coercion claims, which can temper simplistic adoption of PA in legal settings.

In both countries, macro discourse is evolving: there is increasing recognition that PA should be seen through the lens of relational harm and coercive control, not just child choice.

Europe (Spain, Other Nations): Judicial Culture, Gender Norms, and State Intervention

Many European nations occupy an intermediate position between Anglo legal paradigms and civil law traditions. In Spain, for example, the UN has criticised the country's judicial handling of PA and gendered biases in custody matters. In one high-profile case, a court asserted that keeping a child with the mother risked further alienating the father. The UN noted this as a failure of child protection.

In Spain and other parts of Europe, PA is often addressed within child welfare legislation, psychological assessment norms, and domestic violence frameworks rather than as a standalone issue. The macrosystem there includes legal approaches that prioritise harm, gender equity, and child rights, which shape how PA allegations are evaluated and constrained.

In nations such as Sweden, Norway, or Germany, there is also greater scepticism of PA and stronger ethical governance of expert testimony. In Germany, for example, the *German Constitutional Court* recently ruled that the PAS concept cannot serve as a reliable basis for custody decisions, citing a lack of scientific consensus.

These variations demonstrate how macro-level legal culture and professional norms calibrate how PA is recognised, contested, or restricted.

India and China: Collectivist Norms, Hierarchy, and Local Legal Traditions

In countries such as India and China, the macro culture often emphasises familial duty, filial piety, hierarchy, and community cohesion. The macrosystem's normative assumptions about parent–child loyalty, parental authority, and shame may magnify the emotional stakes of separation or defection.

In India, divorce and custody are still heavily influenced by religious laws, patriarchal norms, and family honour. Children "choosing" between parents may be seen very differently: less as individual autonomy and more as betrayal of family unity. PA in India may thus be more likely to be interpreted as rebellion, moral failing, or spiritual deviation rather than as a psychological phenomenon. Legal and familial systems may be slower to recognise PA explicitly, as relational conflict is often handled through informal mediation or family councils.

In China, the state and community play a strong role in family regulation, and family stability is highly prized. The macrosystem places strong emphasis on harmony and social order. In such contexts, overt alienation may be less socially tolerated, but more covert forms may proliferate. The discourse may emphasise "parental responsibility," "family unity," and "filial respect," making it more difficult to name or treat PA as a dysfunction rather than as moral failure.

Because academic and legal recognition of PA is relatively nascent in these contexts, there is often reticence or ambiguity in how courts treat accusations of alienation, and there is less development of specialist professionals or jurisprudence centred on PA. This reflects how the macrosystem's values and institutional priorities suppress or delay the emergence of PA discourse.

Brazil and Latin America: Legislative Recognition, Symbolic Power, and Cultural Contestation

Brazil offers a fascinating case of a macrosystem that has advanced towards formal legislative recognition of what is sometimes called "alienação parental." In Brazil, "alienação parental" (parental alienation) is a legally recognised concept in family law, and courts may apply specific remedies.

However, even in Brazil, the macrosystem remains contested: debates continue about whether the concept is used to undermine protective claims (e.g., in cases of domestic violence) or whether it can be weaponised by controlling parents. Legislative acceptance does not guarantee consistent or sensitive practice; it must contend with local beliefs, power imbalances, gender norms, and judicial capacity.

In Latin America more broadly, the macro discourse includes a tension between paternal rights activism, feminist critiques, and children's rights movements, mirroring similar tensions in the Anglo world but refracted through distinct cultural lenses of family honour, trust, and state paternalism.

Comparative Reflections: How Macro Beliefs Shape PA Presentation and Intervention

From these national examples, several patterns and lessons emerge:

1. Macro frameworks pre-structure what is visible or legitimate. In highly litigious settings (USA), PA is framed as adversarial legal turf; in welfare/institutionally cautious settings (UK, Australia), it is constrained by protective norms; in collectivist societies, it may be interpreted through moral or social lenses; and in legislative contexts (Brazil), it acquires formal status but is still mediated by cultural bias.
2. Cultural beliefs about parenthood, gender, and loyalty matter deeply. Where motherhood is idealised or seen as the default caregiver, accusations of alienation by mothers are treated with scepticism. Where fatherhood is perceived as under threat in public discourse, courts may be more receptive to "father's alienation" claims.
3. The stage of PA discourse reflects macrosystem maturity. Some countries are still in denial or scepticism regarding PA; others are experimenting with cautious use, and others have legislated frameworks. This progression is itself a chronosystem shift within the macrosystem.
4. Macro structures can amplify or contain harm. In countries with strong legal and social protection systems (child welfare agencies, domestic violence enforcement, and co-parenting norms), PA may be more likely to be contested or curtailed. In countries with weak institutional safeguards, PA may flourish undetected or unchallenged.
5. Intervention models must be culturally adapted. A one-size-fits-all model imported from one nation is likely to fail in another. For example, requiring children in China to actively reject one parent may conflict with cultural expectations of filiality; insisting on court-ordered reunification without social supports may backfire in India's hierarchical, extended family systems.

Thus, when we say, "in this country PA is approached thus," that statement is not neutral; it is the product of macro-level beliefs, institutional legacies, legal traditions, and discursive power. Understanding PA must always be a cultural and ideological act, not merely a psychological one.

BIBLIOGRAPHY

Bronfenbrenner, U. (1994). Ecological models of human development. *International Encyclopedia of Education*, 3(2), 37–43.

Korosi, S. (2024). Social alienation in families. In *Advance: A SAGE preprints community* (p. 10). Sage Publishing. https://doi.org/10.31124/advance.171802097.78339306/v1

Korosi, S. (2025a). *Parental alienation: Power, gender, politics and policy in Australia and internationally*. Authorea Preprints.

Korosi, S. (2025b). The end of gendered policy: A new public policy framework for alienation in families (parental alienation). *Advance: A SAGE Preprints Community*, 21.

Korosi, S., & Green, K. (2024). Starting the dialogue on a social and public health policy framework for alienation in families (parental alienation). In *Advance: A SAGE Preprints Community*. Sage Publishing. https://doi.org/10.31124/advance.172162741.19477121/v1

9

PARENTAL ALIENATION AS VIOLENCE

Up to this point, we have examined Parental Alienation (PA) through various lenses: the psychological profiles of those involved, the theoretical models that help us interpret behaviour, and the broader sociocultural systems in which these dynamics unfold. However, if we are to fully grasp the seriousness of PA, we must now turn to the behaviours themselves. What is actually being done, and to what effect? This chapter considers PA as a form of violence, not metaphorically, but in concrete, definable terms that align with existing frameworks in both child protection and family violence discourse.

By mapping alienating behaviours onto established models such as coercive control and psychological child abuse, we can recognise PA not merely as a private family conflict or clinical anomaly but as a pattern of relational harm with clear parallels to other forms of interpersonal violence. The motivations behind alienating behaviour, control, retaliation, and fear of abandonment, are often indistinguishable from those that underpin domestic abuse. Similarly, the emotional impact on children mirrors the long-term consequences of exposure to chronic psychological maltreatment. Recognising PA as violence challenges us to rethink not only how we intervene but how we name, frame, and respond to this deeply damaging phenomenon.

DOI: 10.4324/9781003630944-12

PARENTAL ALIENATION AS A PATTERN OF DOMESTIC/ RELATIONAL VIOLENCE

Rather than a standalone dysfunction, PA often functions as a component within a broader campaign of relational violence. In such cases, the alienating parent does not merely withhold a relationship but actively weaponises the parent–child bond to isolate, disempower, and inflict emotional harm on the targeted parent and the child. When this pattern is sustained, it meets the criteria of abuse in its own right and should be conceptualised as violence – emotional, psychological, and relational.

In practice, alienating parents may deploy tactics such as sustained denigration, false accusations, misrepresentations of the targeted parent, and the cultivation of fear or distrust in the child towards that parent. These strategies mirror classic forms of psychological abuse: manipulation of truth, undermining credibility, inducing guilt or shame, and controlling the emotional environment. In doing so, the alienator undermines the targeted parent's authority, erodes the child's confidence in that parent, and deepens separation, not through neutral estrangement but via coercive harm.

In many jurisdictions, the alienating parent also engages legal or institutional systems as part of their campaign: making spurious abuse or neglect claims, triggering the involvement of child protective services, seeking restraining orders, or contesting visitation under claims of danger. In these acts, the parent uses the veneer of "child protection" or "legal process" to further marginalise the targeted parent, restricting or removing access under the guise of safeguarding. These parallel strategies reinforce the power imbalance and make resistance more difficult for the targeted parent.

When we view PA through this lens, that of relational violence, what appears to some as a custody dispute becomes, at least in high-conflict cases, a persistent, multifaceted assault on relational ties, identity, and emotional safety. Recognising PA as violence emphasises that it is not a peripheral irritant but a serious harmful pattern demanding intervention rooted in both safety and restoration for the child and the parent.

PARENTAL ALIENATION AS COERCIVE CONTROL

Parental alienation often mirrors the tactics and logic of coercive control, a sustained pattern of intimidation, isolation, threats, and manipulation, designed to dominate another's sense of autonomy, agency, and relational integrity. In the domain of PA, the child becomes the instrument through which control is exercised against the targeted parent.

The alienating parent may gaslight the child, subtly planting doubts about the targeted parent's love, reliability, or intentions. They may distort or withhold information, retell past interactions in a biased way, or withhold context, all with the effect of reshaping the child's memory and perception. Over time, this narrative control becomes internalised.

In more extreme instances, the alienator can cultivate an atmosphere of fear by exaggerating the flaws of the targeted parent or suggesting danger or unpredictability. The child is conditioned to believe that rejection is protective. To maintain this illusion, the alienating parent may restrict, monitor, or sabotage contact outright, erasing opportunities for the child to disconfirm the alienating narrative.

Through these tactics, the targeted parent becomes isolated from the child's world, not only physically but emotionally and narratively. The alienating parent dominates the discourse about the child's reality, making it difficult for the targeted parent to reclaim relational presence. This dynamic is precisely what coercive control theorists identify as the erosion of autonomy and the monopolisation of relational space.

Recognising this overlap is critical: it invites us to treat high-level alienation as not just pathological behaviour but as a systemic, controlling campaign, one that must be responded to with the same seriousness we accord to intimate partner or domestic violence cases.

PARENTAL ALIENATION AS PSYCHOLOGICAL ABUSE

Beyond its overlap with coercive control, PA aligns squarely with psychological abuse, particularly in its aim to distort reality and manipulate emotional bonds. The core tactic is relational poison: repeated negative remarks, comparisons, misrepresentations, and emotional triangulation, all designed to degrade the child's trust in the targeted parent.

For example, the alienating parent may repeatedly denigrate the targeted parent in front of the child, "They never cared about you," "They were always too busy for you," to shift the child's appraisal of that parent. They may subtly position themselves as the superior caregiver and portray the other parent as neglectful, insensitive, or even dangerous. Exaggerated or misleading accounts of past events may be used, or selective memories invoked, to paint the targeted parent as untrustworthy.

One particularly insidious tactic is memory manipulation: vying for the child's internal narrative by rewriting or reframing past experiences, often insulating the child from any positive memories of the targeted parent. The alienator may deny or contest the child's recollections, invoking confusion, shame, or self-doubt.

In more advanced cases, gaslighting is leveraged, denying or minimising the child's own experience, inducing emotional self-doubt, or creating a pervasive sense that the child's own memory and feelings are unreliable. The child's internal sense of relational reality becomes fragile, and they may come to distrust their own emotional truth.

When these tactics are systematic, sustained, and relationally embedded, they meet standard definitions of emotional/psychological maltreatment of the child. PA is not just harm to a parental relationship; it is harm to the child's inner world, involving control over perception, memory, and loyalty.

PARENTAL ALIENATION AS POST-SEPARATION ABUSE

Parental alienation is especially harmful because it often continues or intensifies *after* the formal end of a parental relationship. PA is thus a form of post-separation abuse, in which the alienating parent uses the child as a proxy to maintain control, retaliate against the other parent, or regulate their own fear of abandonment.

This abuse takes many forms: limiting or denying access to the targeted parent, making false reports to authorities, or belittling the targeted parent in the child's view. The abuse is often framed as justified, "I'm protecting you," which complicates recognition and response. For the targeted parent, this prolongs wounds, deepens helplessness, and may prevent resolution or closure. For the child, it traps them in a relational cage, torn between loyalty, fear, and confusion.

Understanding PA as post-separation abuse shifts attention from divorce as rupture to continuing relational control. It frames alienation as a continuation, not a cessation, of relational harm and highlights why protective interventions must operate long after separation.

PARENTAL ALIENATION AS CHILD PSYCHOLOGICAL MALTREATMENT

Parental alienation also intersects directly with child abuse frameworks, particularly those addressing psychological maltreatment. In many jurisdictions, emotional abuse is recognised as a legitimate form of child maltreatment, manifested through harm to the child's self-concept, relational capacity, and emotional development. Alienation tactics often fall squarely within these definitions.

In some cases, the alienating parent may even levy false allegations of abuse against the targeted parent, wielding them as tools in the alienation campaign. Whether baseless or legitimate, these allegations must be carefully scrutinised, as they may be defensive, retaliatory, or part of a broader manipulative strategy. Professionals must be vigilant not to automatically dismiss abuse reports but to differentiate true protective concerns from instrumental allegations used to further estrangement.

When experts diagnose PA, they must always contextualise it within an abuse-informed framework, asking whether the child has been emotionally burdened, manipulated, or deprived of relational safety, and whether the alienating narrative has supplanted the child's relational trust. Interventions must aim to restore relational integrity, protect the child's psychological welfare, and reintegrate the targeted parent, while actively safeguarding against further abuse.

PARENTAL ALIENATION AND RELATIONAL CONFLICT ESCALATION THEORY (RCET)

A promising theoretical contribution to understanding violence dynamics in family systems is Relational Conflict Escalation Theory (RCET) by Courtney Dowdall, a model derived from non-cooperative game theory (NCGT) and adapted to intimate and familial relationships. RCET reframes conflict not as isolated incidents of dysfunction but as a sequence of strategic decisions shaped by asymmetrical power, emotional volatility, and constrained options. While initially designed to illuminate patterns in intimate partner violence (IPV), its core insights can be productively applied to the domain of parental alienation, particularly in explaining how relational conflict intensifies over time.

RCET rests on three foundational concepts: (1) leverage asymmetry (formerly referred to as asymmetric power and information); (2) sequential and cumulative interactions; and (3) bounded rationality. These elements collectively describe how one party, often the alienating parent, strategically adapts their behaviour over time to maintain control, while the responding party, commonly the targeted parent, navigates a deteriorating relational terrain marked by shifting threats, diminished autonomy, and escalating harm.

In the context of PA, leverage asymmetry emerges when one parent exercises control not through overt physical violence but through coercive mechanisms such as manipulating the child's perceptions, controlling access, or influencing institutional actors (e.g., schools, courts). The alienating parent's capacity to distort narratives, orchestrate gatekeeping, or use legal delay as a tactic produces an environment of strategic concealment and misinformation. Like IPV perpetrators who signal dominance through threats or surveillance, alienating parents often send credible signals (e.g., threats to seek sole custody or allegations of abuse), which narrow the targeted parent's perceived options and increase the psychological and legal costs of resistance.

Sequential and cumulative interactions are central to how PA unfolds. An initial slight, such as the dissolution of the relationship, may lead to boundary-testing behaviours: subtle denigration of the other parent, obstruction of contact, or triangulation through the child. These behaviours, when met with either compliance or failed challenge, often escalate. For instance, if the targeted parent responds by attempting legal redress, the alienating parent may interpret this as a threat to control and escalate their tactics, making more severe allegations, fabricating narratives of harm, or pressuring the child to reject the other parent. This interactional feedback loop parallels RCET's model of escalating conflict, wherein each move invites a strategic counter-move, often under conditions of distorted perception and high emotional cost.

Bounded rationality in PA contexts is especially salient. Targeted parents frequently operate under extreme emotional strain, legal ambiguity, and fear of making matters worse for the child. Their decisions, whether to confront, withdraw, seek help, or comply, may appear inconsistent, but often reflect adaptive strategies in an environment of chronic coercion. Likewise, alienating parents may escalate not from premeditated malice but from deeply embedded narratives of entitlement, perceived threat, or psychological enmeshment. The recursive nature of their strategies may not be fully conscious but unfold in a pattern of self-reinforcing justification and retaliation.

RCET's contribution lies in providing a sequential, strategic lens to these processes. Rather than viewing PA as a static label or a single act of custodial interference, it enables us to see how conflict escalates in patterned, adaptive ways. Crucially, this model explains why interventions that fail to disrupt the perceived strategic gains of alienation, such as weak enforcement of contact orders or a lack of coordinated institutional response, can inadvertently reinforce the alienating parent's behaviour, raising the likelihood of continued or intensified alienation.

Just as in cases of IPV, PA escalation is rarely linear and often path-dependent. The earlier a pattern of control is established and left unchallenged, the more likely it is to evolve into entrenched alienation. Similarly, the longer the child is exposed to these dynamics, the more costly and difficult it becomes for them to reintegrate the alienated parent into their relational world.

In short, RCET extends the violence paradigm of PA by offering a mechanistic account of how alienating behaviours escalate, not merely as expressions of dysfunction but as strategic responses in high-conflict, power-laden relational systems. It aligns with the broader theoretical shift advocated in this chapter: one that positions parental alienation not simply as a contentious custody issue but as a form of relational violence grounded in coercion, asymmetry, and the erosion of relational agency.

IMPLICATIONS FOR PRACTICE AND INTERVENTION

Recognising PA within established frameworks of violence, coercive control, psychological abuse, post-separation abuse, and child maltreatment has profound implications for clinical, legal, and policy-oriented responses. It shifts the focus from custody disputes or high-conflict dynamics to a pattern of relational harm, often requiring urgent, multi-layered intervention. Practitioners must move beyond binary thinking, of favoured versus rejected parent, and instead engage with PA as a complex form of family violence embedded in systems of control, trauma, and institutional response.

Comprehensive, Abuse-Informed Assessment

Professionals must undertake holistic, trauma-informed assessments that evaluate the entire family system. This includes:

- Mapping the family's relational history, patterns of care, separation events, and narratives presented by each party.
- Identifying whether the child's rejection stems from authentic estrangement (e.g., due to abuse) or is indicative of manipulative influence.
- Screening for co-occurring abuse: intimate partner violence, child maltreatment, coercive control, or administrative misuse of systems.

Importantly, assessments should avoid pathologising normal responses to distress, while remaining alert to patterns that clearly indicate alienation rooted in control and harm.

Cross-Disciplinary Collaboration

Effective intervention requires integrated practice across disciplines – family courts, mental health services, social care, and legal representatives. No single agency or profession can adequately address the complexity of PA. Collaborative frameworks ensure:

- Shared language and conceptual clarity across professions.
- Child-focused coordination, with an emphasis on safety, developmental needs, and relational restoration.
- Integrated safety planning that considers all members of the family, particularly where there are ongoing risks from domestic violence or coercive control.

Ongoing Therapeutic Support

Alienation is rarely resolved through legal means alone. Sustained progress requires:

- Long-term relational work to rebuild trust, repair attachment injuries, and deconstruct internalised narratives of rejection.
- Support for the alienating parent (where safe and appropriate) to address their own attachment trauma, maladaptive beliefs, or personality vulnerabilities.
- Community or peer group support for targeted parents and children, reducing isolation and validating their experiences.

Recognition of Legal and Administrative Abuse

In cases where PA is compounded by misuse of legal systems, professionals must recognise this as a form of administrative coercion. This includes:

- False allegations weaponised in court to remove access.
- Strategic litigation to delay, exhaust, or financially burden the targeted parent.
- Manipulation of child protection procedures to instigate unwarranted interventions.

Courts and child protection agencies must be trained to distinguish between genuine safeguarding concerns and strategic abuse of process, developing safeguards to prevent institutional complicity in alienation.

Reaffirming the Child's Best Interests

Across all interventions, the wellbeing of the child must remain paramount. This involves:

- Recognising that both alienation and exposure to family violence are developmentally harmful.
- Ensuring that decisions prioritise long-term relational stability, safety, and the child's right to authentic, unmanipulated connection with both parents wherever possible.
- Avoiding short-term fixes (e.g., default shared care) in situations where PA is masking deeper psychological control or abuse.

SUMMARY

This chapter reframes PA not merely as a psychological or relational issue but as a form of violence with clear parallels to established models of domestic abuse, coercive control, and child psychological maltreatment. Building on prior chapters that explored theoretical, individual, and contextual dimensions, this chapter interrogates the *actions* at the core of PA and their devastating consequences.

It argues that PA is often part of a broader pattern of relational and post-separation abuse, wherein the alienating parent uses the child as a tool to exert control over, or emotionally harm, the targeted parent. Tactics such as denigration, gaslighting, memory manipulation, and the strategic use of legal or institutional systems are examined in detail. These behaviours are mapped onto frameworks such as coercive control and emotional abuse, highlighting how PA functions as a sustained campaign of isolation, domination, and narrative control.

The chapter also identifies PA as a form of child psychological maltreatment, noting that the child is not merely a passive participant but a direct victim of manipulation that distorts their sense of reality, emotional safety, and relational security. It emphasises that professionals must recognise this abuse not only as interpersonal harm but as institutionally reinforced when courts or services are manipulated to restrict access under false pretences.

BIBLIOGRAPHY

Berman, P. W., & Weisinger, E. (2022). Parental alienation vs coercive control: Controversial issues and current research. *Journal of Family Trauma, Child Custody & Child Development*. https://doi.org/10.1080/26904586.2022.2125475

Dowdall, C. M., Lysova, A., & Hine, B. A. (2026). *Escalation and exclusion: Fathers' narratives of navigating noncooperation and the dynamics of parental alienation*. Manuscript Submitted for Publication.

Harman, J. J., Kruk, E., & Hines, D. A. (2018). Parental alienating behaviors: An unacknowledged form of family violence. *Psychological Bulletin*, *144*, 1275–1299. https://doi.org/10.1037/bul0000175

Isailă, O. M., & Hostiuc, S. (2022). Medical-legal and psychosocial considerations on parental alienation as a form of child abuse: A brief review. *Healthcare*, *10*, 1134. https://doi.org/10.3390/healthcare10061134

Kruk, E. (2018). Parental alienation as a form of emotional child abuse: Current state of knowledge and future directions for research. *Family Science Review*, *22*, 141–162.

Kruk, E., & Harman, J. J. (2025). Countering arguments against parental alienation as a form of family violence and child abuse. *The American Journal of Family Therapy*, *53*(2), 117–146. https://doi.org/10.1080/01926187.2024.2396279

Lysova, A., Hanson, K., & Hines, D. A. (2023). "How can I be a victim when I have children?" Abused men's perceptions of their children's exposure to domestic violence. *Journal of Aggression, Maltreatment & Trauma*, *33*(1), 67–84. https://doi.org/10.1080/10926771.2023.2186300

Mercer, J. (2021). Critiquing assumptions about parental alienation: Part 1. The analogy with family violence. *Journal of Family Trauma, Child Custody & Child Development*, 1–17. https://doi.org/10.1080/26904586.2021.1957057

Milchman, M. S. (2021). Distinguishing parental alienation from child abuse and adverse parenting. In *Challenging parental alienation* (pp. 107–137). Routledge.

Rowlands, G. A., Warshak, R. A., & Harman, J. J. (2023). Abused and rejected: The link between intimate partner violence and parental alienation. *Partner Abuse*, *14*(1). http://dx.doi.org/10.1891/PA-2022-0001

Sharples, A. E., Harman, J. J., & Lorandos, D. (2025). Findings of abuse in families affected by parental alienation. *Journal of Family Violence*, *40*(2), 225–235. https://doi.org/10.1007/s10896-023-00575-x

von Boch-Galhau, W. (2021). Parental alienation: A serious form of child psychological abuse that affects children all over the world. *Highlights on Medicine and Medical Science*, *3*, 127–137. https://doi.org/10.9734/bpi/hmms/v3/9041D

PART 3

WHAT IS THE IMPACT?

10

IMPACT ON CHILDREN

Parental alienation is not merely a transient disruption in a child's family life; it is a profound relational trauma with enduring consequences. This chapter examines the far-reaching effects of the alienation process on children, highlighting how its psychological and emotional toll often extends well beyond childhood into adolescence, adulthood, and even intergenerational relationships. Alienated children may experience identity confusion, attachment disruption, and internalised guilt, all of which can manifest in long-term mental health challenges, academic difficulties, impaired social functioning, and compromised future relationships. Crucially, these impacts do not emerge in isolation; they are shaped by the sustained and coercive nature of the alienating behaviours to which children are exposed. By exploring these effects in depth, this chapter highlights the urgent need for early identification and intervention, not only to resolve immediate family conflict but also to prevent the lasting developmental scars that alienation can inflict.

EMOTIONAL AND PSYCHOLOGICAL EFFECTS

Parental alienation (PA) exerts profound emotional and psychological harm on children, often disrupting their developmental trajectory in ways that can persist well into adulthood. Far beyond the immediate distress of parental conflict, PA can function as a sustained psychological injury that affects a child's identity, sense of safety, and capacity for emotional regulation.

DOI: 10.4324/9781003630944-14

Loss of Attachment and Identity Disruption

Children subjected to parental alienating behaviours often lose not only a parent but also a crucial aspect of their personal identity. The severing of the relationship with a once-loved parent can lead to confusion about one's own self-worth, values, and family history. This identity disturbance is compounded by the inability to process or healthily grieve these losses, particularly when the alienation is not addressed. For many children, this results in disenfranchised and unresolved grief, which can linger into adolescence and adulthood.

Depression and Anxiety

A growing body of empirical research demonstrates a strong association between PA and internalising symptoms such as depression and anxiety. Recent longitudinal studies in Chinese adolescent populations (see work by Wang et al.) have shown that exposure to alienating behaviours significantly predicts depressive symptoms and broader emotional distress. These effects are often mediated by disrupted attachment and diminished self-esteem, and further exacerbated by impaired emotion regulation strategies such as poor cognitive reappraisal and reliance on suppression.

Emotional Dysregulation and Mental Health Risk

Alienated children frequently exhibit difficulties with emotional regulation, including heightened reactivity, passivity, or emotional constriction. As PA fundamentally damages the parent–child attachment, adolescents subsequently struggle with managing emotions effectively, leading to increased risk for both internalising (e.g., depression, anxiety) and externalising problems (e.g., aggression, rule-breaking behaviour).

Self-Esteem Distortion

Low self-esteem is a common consequence of PA, particularly when children internalise the alienating parent's negative portrayal of the targeted parent. This internalisation can lead children to question their own worth, develop pervasive self-doubt, or adopt distorted views of reality and relationships. In some cases, children may also develop an inflated or omnipotent sense of self as a defence mechanism against the psychological dissonance caused by the loss of a valued caregiver.

Conflict of Loyalty and Cognitive Distortions

One of the most painful psychological burdens for alienated children is the continuous management of the induced conflict of loyalty. The fear of abandonment or emotional withdrawal by the alienating parent leads children to suppress their affection for the targeted parent, even in the absence of any abusive behaviour. Over time, this coerced alignment results in black-and-white thinking, false memories, and inconsistent or illogical narratives about the alienated parent, all of which impair critical thinking and interpersonal functioning.

ACADEMIC AND SOCIAL OUTCOMES

The consequences of parental alienation (PA) extend well beyond the psychological domain, significantly affecting children's functioning in academic settings and social environments. As children navigate the complex emotional terrain of loyalty conflicts, psychological manipulation, and family disintegration, their ability to engage in learning and build healthy peer relationships is often severely compromised.

Disruption of Academic Functioning

Children exposed to PA frequently struggle to maintain focus and motivation in educational contexts. The ongoing emotional strain, characterised by anxiety, sadness, confusion, and internalised guilt, can impair cognitive processes essential for learning, such as attention, memory consolidation, and executive functioning. As such, alienated children are more likely to exhibit poor academic performance, stemming from emotional exhaustion, reduced self-efficacy, and persistent preoccupation with familial conflict. Moreover, absenteeism is often more common in these children, whether due to psychosomatic illness (e.g., headaches, stomach pain) or lack of motivation, further compounding academic disengagement.

Impaired Peer Relationships

Alienated children may also experience significant difficulties forming and sustaining peer relationships. Emotional dysregulation, identity confusion, and diminished self-worth can manifest as social withdrawal, overdependence on peers, or maladaptive interpersonal behaviours. For some children, the alienating parent may actively or subtly discourage socialisation with peers as a means of exerting further control, leading to isolation and a breakdown of age-appropriate social development. These interpersonal deficits are not merely transient; they can lay the foundation for long-term relational dysfunction extending into adulthood.

Vulnerability to Bullying and Victimisation

Several studies, including longitudinal research from Wang et al., underscore the increased vulnerability of alienated children to peer victimisation.

The combination of low self-esteem, emotional fragility, and impaired emotion regulation may make these children more susceptible to bullying. Additionally, children who exhibit signs of psychological distress, such as hyper-reactivity, social awkwardness, or excessive need for approval, may be perceived as "different" by peers, increasing the likelihood of being targeted. Lacking the social confidence and resilience typically fostered in stable family environments, these children often struggle to assert boundaries or seek support when confronted with hostile peer dynamics.

Distorted Social Norms and Behaviour

Alienated children often internalise distorted views of authority, trust, and interpersonal conduct, shaped by the manipulative narratives of the alienating parent. This may result in behaviours that violate social norms, such as aggression, dishonesty, or manipulative peer interactions. In some cases, children may model the alienating parent's behaviours, including coercion, rejection, or scapegoating, in their own peer relationships. Such patterns further reinforce social rejection or instability, contributing to a self-perpetuating cycle of dysfunction. They are also more likely to engage in maladaptive behaviours such as substance use, self-harm, or premature sexual activity. These developmental disruptions mirror the effects seen in other forms of child maltreatment and underscore the necessity of conceptualising PA as a form of psychological abuse.

Compromised Social Learning

Because PA frequently disrupts one of the child's primary attachment relationships, opportunities for learning core social-emotional competencies, such as empathy, reciprocity, conflict resolution, and emotional expression, may be lost or distorted. These deficits not only impede current peer interactions but also affect the broader developmental trajectory of social integration, including future friendships, romantic relationships, and workplace functioning.

LONG-TERM EFFECTS AND ADULT RELATIONSHIPS

The psychological and relational damage caused by parental alienation (PA) rarely ends in childhood. Instead, the unresolved trauma and disrupted developmental processes associated with PA frequently persist into adulthood, shaping the individual's capacity to engage in secure, trusting, and reciprocal relationships. Adult children of alienation often describe their experience as a form of "relational haunting," a residual echo of childhood betrayal and confusion that continues to interfere with emotional stability, attachment formation, and identity development.

Erosion of Relational Trust

Many adults who experienced PA as children struggle with a pervasive mistrust of others. The experience of being manipulated into rejecting a once-loved parent, often accompanied by false narratives and psychological pressure, can undermine the individual's foundational sense of relational safety. As a result, they may approach friendships, romantic partnerships, or even professional interactions with guardedness or suspicion, fearing vulnerability will lead to further betrayal or abandonment.

Barriers to Emotional Intimacy

The long-standing impact of emotional suppression, role-reversal dynamics, or enmeshment with the alienating parent can create enduring difficulties with emotional openness. Adult survivors may find it challenging to express vulnerability, regulate emotional responses in conflict, or tolerate ambiguity in relationships; these are essential factors for establishing and maintaining intimacy. These challenges are not merely psychological in nature; they are often embodied, showing up in patterns of withdrawal, over-control, or emotional disconnection.

Intergenerational Transmission of Dysfunction

One of the more troubling legacies of PA is the risk of intergenerational repetition. Without recognition or therapeutic intervention, adult survivors may unconsciously replicate relational dynamics from their childhood, either by entering into controlling or manipulative relationships themselves, or by enacting alienating behaviours in conflict with co-parents. In some cases, the internalised schema of loyalty conflicts, black-and-white thinking, or emotional suppression can lead to the very same dynamics they once suffered as children being perpetuated with their own children or partners.

Persistent Mental Health Challenges

The long-term psychological burden of PA often includes chronic symptoms of depression, anxiety, identity confusion, and, in more severe cases, post-traumatic stress disorder (PTSD). Unlike situational trauma, PA-related distress tends to be insidious, embedded within the child's core developmental years. This makes it harder to identify, treat, or even acknowledge in adulthood, as the symptoms often appear diffuse or are misattributed to other life stressors.

Delayed Grief and Existential Loss

Many adult children of PA experience a deep, often disenfranchised grief when they come to recognise what was lost; not only a relationship with a parent, but also time, identity, and formative emotional experiences. In cases where contact is re-established with the alienated parent, the relationship may remain fragile, overshadowed by unresolved guilt, shame, or confusion. For others, the "awakening" to having been manipulated can also destabilise relationships with the alienating parent, leading to secondary losses and emotional upheaval.

Strained Parental Bonds in Adulthood

Even when physical reunification occurs, emotional repair can be elusive. Long-standing alienation often leaves both the targeted parent and adult child unsure of how to relate to each other. The years of lost trust, distorted memories, and unresolved trauma can make it difficult to rebuild a mutually secure and emotionally available bond. Similarly, re-evaluating the relationship with the alienating parent may provoke a crisis of identity or loyalty, particularly if the realisation occurs without therapeutic support.

ADULTIFICATION AND PARENTIFICATION

One of the more insidious effects of parental alienation (PA) lies in its capacity to invert regular developmental roles, forcing children into premature psychological and emotional adulthood. This phenomenon, commonly referred to as *adultification*, occurs when children are expected to assume responsibilities, make decisions, and bear emotional burdens that exceed their developmental readiness. It is a hallmark of dysfunctional family systems and is particularly prevalent in alienating environments where power dynamics are distorted and emotional boundaries are blurred.

Premature Role Assumption

In PA contexts, children are often subtly or overtly recruited into the psychological world of the alienating parent. Rather than being protected from adult concerns, they are exposed to the complexities of legal disputes, narratives of betrayal, and emotionally charged judgements about the other parent. In some cases, they are asked to make decisions about contact, testify in court, or express opinions about matters far beyond their developmental capacity. This premature engagement in adult roles not only compromises the child's emotional safety but also impairs their ability to explore age-appropriate tasks such as play, identity formation, and peer bonding.

Emotional Parentification

Emotional parentification often emerges as a direct consequence of *enmeshment* (as described in Chapter 7), a process in which psychological boundaries between parent and child become blurred or entirely collapsed. In alienating family systems, enmeshment often serves as a strategy for maintaining control and allegiance, with emotional parentification being one of its key mechanisms. The child is not merely emotionally close to the alienating parent; they are psychologically fused with them, recruited into the parent's inner world, and burdened with emotional responsibilities that far exceed their developmental capacity. Rather than receiving nurturing and guidance, the child becomes a confidant, caretaker, or emotional surrogate, consoling the parent, validating their grievances, and, at times, absorbing their anger or pain. This fusion of roles undermines the child's autonomy and identity development, as their self-worth becomes contingent upon stabilising the emotional state of the parent. Over time, this dynamic instils a chronic sense of guilt, emotional over-responsibility, and confusion around relational roles, leaving the child ill-equipped for healthy attachment and emotional reciprocity in adulthood.

In the context of PA, the alienating parent may leverage this parentified relationship to solidify the child's alliance further and intensify the rejection of the targeted parent. The child, positioned as an emotional protector or surrogate partner, may feel that any affection shown towards the alienated parent is a betrayal of the parent who "needs" them. This dynamic not only entrenches the alienation but also burdens the child with impossible emotional conflicts that may persist unresolved into adulthood.

Undermining of Attachment and Autonomy

At its core, adultification disrupts the natural hierarchy of caregiving and attachment. When children are required to meet the emotional needs of a parent, especially in the absence of the protective buffering that a healthy relationship with the targeted parent might have provided, they lose the psychological space to develop autonomy, emotional regulation, and a coherent sense of self. This developmental interference is not temporary; it reconfigures the trajectory of their relational templates, often with lasting effects on their ability to form and maintain healthy adult relationships.

Developmental and Relational Costs

The consequences of adultification and parentification in the context of PA are thus far-reaching. These children may appear prematurely mature, compliant, or overly responsible; traits often misinterpreted as resilience. In reality, they are coping strategies born of survival in an emotionally coercive environment. Over time, these children are more likely to develop anxiety disorders, perfectionism, chronic guilt, and difficulties establishing appropriate boundaries in future relationships. Moreover, they may struggle with self-care, emotional dependency, or even reproduce similar dynamics in their own parenting or partnerships.

LOSSES TO THE CHILD

Children subjected to PA experience a complex web of losses that extends far beyond the severance of a relationship with one parent. These are not isolated incidents of grief but layered, interrelated deprivations that shape the child's developing sense of self, family, and place in the world.

Loss of a Coherent Sense of Self

Perhaps the most insidious loss is the diminishment of the child's individual identity. As mentioned above, in rejecting the alienated parent, the child often feels compelled to repudiate aspects of themselves that are associated with that parent, genetic, temperamental, or relational. This rejection is not freely chosen but instead shaped through enmeshment and loyalty conflicts orchestrated by the alienating parent. As a result, the child becomes increasingly dependent on the alienating parent for identity and validation, suppressing independent thought and expression in the process. This compromised selfhood may manifest later as chronic low self-esteem, identity diffusion, and internalised shame.

Loss of Childhood and Developmental Opportunities

Alienated children are frequently deprived of normative childhood experiences. Time that should be spent in play, education, and exploration is instead consumed by emotional labour, such as managing the alienating parent's distress, navigating divided loyalties, and avoiding punishments for perceived disloyalty. Processes described above, such as *adultification, emotional parentification*, and even *infantilisation,* undermine the child's opportunity to develop autonomy, resilience, and age-appropriate social skills. Retrospectively, many alienated individuals describe their childhood as prematurely ended, devoid of innocence, safety, or play.

Loss of a "Good Enough" Parent

Through the systematic corruption of reality, the alienated parent, who was previously a safe and loving figure, is recharacterised as dangerous, rejecting, or unloving. This distorted narrative is absorbed by the child, who comes to believe it as truth, often denying any positive memories or feelings associated with that parent. The psychological loss is profound: the child loses not only a parent but also the capacity to grieve that loss authentically. What is mourned is not just the absence of a relationship but the erasure of a once-secure attachment.

Loss of Extended Family and Social Capital

Alienation often leads to the severance of ties with the extended family on the targeted parent's side, grandparents, aunts, uncles, and cousins, who are typically perceived as "extensions" of the rejected parent. These individuals offer not just emotional support but also cultural identity, traditions, knowledge, and opportunities. Losing them limits the child's access to social capital and relational networks that foster wellbeing and connectedness. It is a loss that is both immediate and cumulative.

Loss of Community and Belonging

In some cases, PABs include relocation, either within the country or internationally, which functions to further isolate the child from not only the alienated parent but also friends, schools, cultural traditions, and broader community anchors. This compounds the child's sense of alienation and instability, removing external sources of validation and continuity. The child is often left to navigate these dislocations without recognition or support, deepening their emotional solitude.

IMPACT ON PHYSICAL HEALTH

Parental alienation (PA) is often understood primarily through a psychological lens; however, its impact extends somatically, influencing a child's physiological development and physical health. The toxic stress induced by prolonged exposure to alienating behaviours functions not merely as an emotional burden but as a sustained physiological threat that dysregulates the body's core stress-response systems.

Chronic Activation of the Stress Response

When children are repeatedly subjected to parental conflict, emotional manipulation, or enforced rejection of a caregiver, their stress-response systems, particularly the hypothalamic–pituitary–adrenal (HPA) axis, are likely to be chronically activated. While acute stress responses are adaptive in short-term situations, chronic activation in early life has been associated with a range of detrimental health outcomes, including immune dysregulation, inflammation, and elevated cardiovascular risk. This kind of sustained physiological stress, sometimes termed *toxic stress*, can have lasting effects on brain architecture, metabolic function, and overall health trajectories across the lifespan.

Somatic Symptoms and Functional Disorders

A significant number of children exposed to PA present with somatic complaints that have no clear organic origin. Headaches, gastrointestinal distress, chronic fatigue, and generalised body pain are among the most commonly reported symptoms. These physical manifestations often reflect internalised emotional turmoil, emerging in the body when the child lacks the psychological or relational resources to process stress consciously. In some cases, these somatic symptoms are misdiagnosed or dismissed, obscuring the psychological trauma at their root.

Sleep Disruption and Neurodevelopmental Impact

Sleep disturbance is another prevalent consequence of PA-related stress. Children may suffer from insomnia, frequent nightmares, or disrupted sleep cycles, often linked to hypervigilance or anxiety. Poor sleep not only impairs daytime functioning and academic engagement but also interferes with key neurodevelopmental processes, such as memory consolidation, emotional regulation, and executive functioning. Over time, sleep deprivation can compound the psychological burden and increase vulnerability to mood disorders.

Eating Disturbances and Metabolic Dysregulation

Chronic emotional stress associated with PA can lead to disrupted eating patterns, including loss of appetite, emotional overeating, or irregular meal consumption. In some cases, this contributes to the development of eating disorders or long-term metabolic imbalances such as obesity, insulin resistance, or gastrointestinal disorders. These effects are particularly concerning in the context of childhood and adolescence, when growth and hormonal regulation are highly sensitive to environmental stressors.

Increased Risk for Chronic Illness

Longitudinal research into adverse childhood experiences (ACEs), which PA is increasingly being recognised as, has consistently linked early relational trauma with heightened risk for chronic health conditions later in life. These include cardiovascular disease, autoimmune disorders, diabetes, and even early mortality. The mechanisms are complex but are believed to involve prolonged inflammation, epigenetic changes, and health-risk behaviours adopted as coping strategies in adolescence or adulthood.

THE ROLE OF GENDER IN PARENTAL ALIENATION

Gender plays a complex and often underexplored role in how parental alienation (PA) unfolds, is experienced by children, and is interpreted by society and professional systems. Both the gender of the child and the alienating parent influence the manifestation, recognition, and consequences of PA, shaped not only by psychological dynamics but also by sociocultural expectations regarding masculinity, femininity, and parenting roles.

Gendered Expressions of Emotional Distress

Children of different genders may exhibit divergent responses to the emotional disruption and psychological stress caused by PA. Boys, for instance, are more likely to externalise their distress through aggression, defiance, or acting-out behaviours, responses that may be misinterpreted as conduct disorders rather than signs of trauma. These behaviours can obscure the underlying cause of their suffering and lead to punitive rather than therapeutic interventions. Girls, conversely, are statistically more prone to internalising disorders in response to alienation-related stress, including anxiety, depression, and disordered eating. Such symptoms are often pathologised in isolation, without recognition of their relational roots.

Exposure to Alienating Behaviours

Recent empirical data has complicated prior assumptions about gender symmetry in PA experiences. Notably, emerging research shows that male adults are statistically more likely to report having been exposed to parental alienating behaviours (PABs) during childhood than female adults. While the reasons for this discrepancy remain under investigation, possible explanations include gender differences in reporting, recall, socialisation, or the types of alienating strategies used. This finding challenges older assumptions that PA primarily affects mothers as targeted parents and invites a re-evaluation of how gender dynamics are conceptualised in both research and practice.

SUMMARY

Parental alienation (PA) represents a serious form of relational trauma that affects children across multiple developmental domains. Far from being a mere by-product of high-conflict separation, PA involves sustained psychological manipulation that erodes a child's emotional well-being, identity formation, and relational stability.

Children exposed to parental alienating behaviours suffer not only emotional distress, such as anxiety, depression, and chronic guilt, but also significant cognitive and behavioural consequences. They may experience difficulties with emotional regulation, self-esteem, and reality testing. Socially and academically, many show signs of disengagement, peer difficulties, or maladaptive coping strategies. These impacts are compounded by physical symptoms such as sleep disturbance, somatic complaints, and increased long-term health risks associated with chronic stress.

Developmentally, PA often leads to role reversals in which children become emotionally responsible for a parent, a process driven by enmeshment. These dynamics can compromise the child's autonomy and undermine their ability to form secure, independent identities. In adulthood, unresolved trauma may manifest as relational dysfunction, internalised shame, or the replication of alienation patterns with future partners or children. Children affected by PA also endure profound losses: of a parent, extended family, stability, and their sense of self. These losses often go unrecognised by others, resulting in disenfranchised grief that is hard to process or resolve.

Professionals must, thus, recognise PA as a form of psychological maltreatment with serious developmental consequences. Early signs, such as emotional role reversal, rigid narratives about a parent, or unexplained distress, require careful assessment and should not be dismissed as typical responses to divorce. Therefore, early multidisciplinary intervention is critical. Fundamentally, PA should be treated as a public health issue, given its clear associations with adverse childhood experiences and lifelong consequences for mental and physical health.

BIBLIOGRAPHY

Excell, H., & Pokhriyal, S. (2024). *Adult alienated children's experience of grief and loss*. Thesis, University of Tasmania. https://doi.org/10.25959/25711311.v1

Harman, J. J., Matthewson, M., & Baker, A. J. L. (2022). Losses experienced by children alienated from a parent. *Current Opinion in Psychology*, *43*, 7–12. https://doi.org/10.1016/j.copsyc.2021.05.002

Miralles, P., Godoy, C., & Hidalgo, M. D. (2021). Long-term emotional consequences of parental alienation exposure in children of divorced parents: A systematic review. *Current Psychology*. https://doi.org/10.1007/s12144-021-02537-2

Verhaar, S., Matthewson, M., & Bentley, C. (2022). The impact of parental alienating behaviours on the mental health of adults alienated in childhood. *Children*, 9, 475. https://doi.org/10.3390/children9040475

Verrocchio, M. C., Baker, A. J. L., & Marchetti, D. (2018). Adult report of childhood exposure to parental alienation at different developmental time periods. *Journal of Family Therapy*, *40*, 602–618. https://doi.org/10.1111/1467-6427.12192

Verrocchio, M. C., Marchetti, D., Carrozzino, D., Compare, A., & Fulcheri, M. (2019). Depression and quality of life in adults perceiving exposure to parental alienation behaviors. *Health and Quality of Life Outcomes*, *17*. https://doi.org/10.1186/s12955-019-1080-6

Wang, K., Huang, Y., Zhang, X., & Wang, X. (2025a). Parental alienation behaviors and adolscent mental health: A two-year longitudinal investigation of parent-child attachment and emotion regulation. *Applied Research in Quality of Life*. https://doi.org/10.1007/s11482-025-10474-6

Wang, K., Lin, B., Huang, Y., & Zhang, X. (2025b). Pathways from parental alienation to adolescent problem behaviors: A longitudinal study of parent-child attachment and emotion regulation. *Children and Youth Services Review*, *172*, 108209. https://doi.org/10.1016/j.childyouth.2025.108209

Wang, K., Xie, X., Zhang, T., Liu, F., Huang, Y., & Zhang, X. (2024). Change brings new life: The influence of parental alienating behaviors on adolescent depression. *Current Psychology*, *43*, 7745–7757. https://doi.org/10.1007/s12144-023-04973-8

11

IMPACT ON TARGETED PARENTS

This chapter explores the profound and multifaceted impact of parental alienation (PA) on targeted parents. While much of the discourse rightly centres on the child's experience, the effects on parents, emotional, psychological, relational, and legal, are no less significant. As we examine the cascading consequences of being unjustly severed from one's child, it becomes evident that PA disrupts not only the parent–child bond but also the very fabric of the targeted parent's identity, well-being, and social standing.

PSYCHOLOGICAL AND EMOTIONAL IMPACT

The psychological impact of PA on the targeted parent is profound and often enduring. While the child is the immediate focus of the alienating behaviours, the emotional fallout for the rejected parent constitutes a severe and frequently overlooked form of psychological harm. The experience is marked by a profound sense of disempowerment, invalidation, and grief, echoing the effects observed in survivors of coercive control.

Psychological Crisis

Being unjustly rejected by one's child, especially when that rejection is sudden, uncharacteristic, or clearly inconsistent with a previously loving bond, can generate a psychological crisis for the targeted parent. This rupture is

DOI: 10.4324/9781003630944-15

often accompanied by intense feelings of helplessness and despair, particularly as the parent witnesses their child adopt hostile or indifferent behaviours that do not originate organically but are shaped by the alienating parent's influence. The emotional toll can mirror that of bereavement, but with the added complexity that the child is still physically present in the world, yet psychologically unreachable. Many targeted parents describe this as a form of "ambiguous loss," a grieving process that lacks both closure and social recognition.

Isolation and Self-Doubt

Feelings of isolation are also pervasive. The stigma associated with being rejected by one's child, especially in the absence of substantiated wrongdoing, can lead parents to withdraw from social networks or avoid disclosing their situation for fear of being misunderstood. This is compounded by a widespread societal tendency to assume that if a child refuses contact, the parent must have done something to deserve it. This kind of misattribution not only invalidates the parent's suffering but can also intensify self-doubt, guilt, and shame. Many begin to question their own parenting, wondering if they are somehow to blame, even when the evidence strongly suggests otherwise.

Secondary Victimisation

Compounding these emotional harms is the frequent experience of *secondary victimisation* through institutional systems, especially family courts. When a parent's grief, frustration, or distress is pathologised, and interpreted not as a consequence of alienation but as its cause, this constitutes a form of blame reversal. Rather than receiving validation or support, targeted parents may be further marginalised by judicial processes that misread protective behaviours as hostility or emotional instability.

Ultimately, the psychological cost of PA is not limited to the temporary pain of estrangement. It disrupts a parent's core identity, erodes their trust in systems meant to protect children, and often leaves lasting emotional scars. The loss is not just of a relationship but of a vital life role, parenthood itself, rendered inaccessible by manipulation, institutional failure, and unresolved grief.

MENTAL HEALTH AND SUICIDE IDEATION

The psychological toll of parental alienation (PA) on targeted parents is not only profound, but it can also be life-threatening. For some, the emotional and relational trauma of being unjustly severed from a child can escalate into severe mental health crises, including clinical depression and suicidal ideation. These outcomes are not rare anomalies; they represent the extreme end of a spectrum of distress caused by prolonged alienation, institutional invalidation, and the erosion of hope.

Depression and Anxiety

Among the most commonly reported psychological consequences are symptoms of depression and anxiety. These may include persistent sadness, hopelessness, sleep disturbances, panic attacks, and overwhelming stress, often exacerbated by the unpredictability of court proceedings, the absence of clear resolution, and the fear of long-term estrangement. In more severe cases, parents may experience trauma-related symptoms such as emotional numbing, hypervigilance, intrusive thoughts, and even suicidal ideation. These are not merely reactions to separation but responses to the *relational betrayal* and sustained psychological invalidation that PA entails.

Ambiguous Grief

The experience of PA involves a unique and deeply complex form of grief. Targeted parents are often forced to endure the psychological pain of losing a child who is still alive while being simultaneously vilified and denied contact. This is a form of ambiguous loss that precludes traditional mourning and complicates emotional processing. The result is often a prolonged state of despair, marked by helplessness, guilt, self-doubt, and, in some cases, clinical depression. These emotional responses are not pathological in themselves; they are rational reactions to sustained relational trauma and perceived injustice.

Suicide Ideation

Among the most alarming consequences of this despair is an elevated risk of suicide. Although empirical research is still emerging, clinical reports and qualitative studies increasingly highlight suicidal ideation among alienated parents, particularly when avenues for legal recourse are exhausted or when they feel disbelieved and unsupported. Suicide risk is exacerbated by a combination of chronic emotional pain, social isolation, legal disempowerment, and perceived or actual failure in their parental role, a role often central to their identity.

Gendered Effects

The mental health burden of PA is especially acute for men. Gendered norms around emotional expression and help-seeking continue to discourage many fathers from acknowledging their distress or accessing mental health support. Societal expectations of stoicism, combined with structural disadvantages in custody decisions, place many men in a psychologically untenable position.

The sense of being both legally marginalised and emotionally silenced compounds their suffering, often leaving them without meaningful outlets for grief or support. These gendered pressures are not merely theoretical; they contribute directly to increased suicide vulnerability among alienated fathers, as highlighted in recent clinical commentary and advocacy literature.

Despite gradual shifts in public discourse recognising the importance of fathers in caregiving roles, institutional and cultural biases persist. Fathers who express distress may be dismissed as controlling, angry, or emotionally unstable, while mothers in similar situations may be met with sympathy. These double standards not only distort the perception of emotional suffering but also actively discourage help-seeking, deepening the risk of psychological collapse.

THE RELATIONSHIP WITH THE CHILD

One of the most profound and enduring consequences of PA is the rupture of the parent–child relationship. For targeted parents, the emotional injury is not simply the loss of contact but the erosion of a once-secure attachment, often replaced by hostility, fear, or emotional detachment from their child. The effects of this rupture are far-reaching, impacting not only the present relationship but also future attempts at repair and reconnection.

Strained Communication

Communication between the targeted parent and the alienated child often becomes strained or entirely severed. Even when contact is maintained, interactions may be marked by tension, emotional withdrawal, or performative compliance. The child may avoid eye contact, refuse to engage in conversation, or respond with monosyllabic answers, making it extremely difficult for the parent to sustain a meaningful emotional connection. These communication barriers are not natural developments of adolescence or separation; they are often the result of subtle (or overt) conditioning by the alienating parent, designed to delegitimise the targeted parent's role and emotional relevance.

Loss of Trust

Trust, a cornerstone of any healthy relationship, is frequently one of the first casualties of alienation. As the child internalises the narrative that the targeted parent is untrustworthy, dangerous, or emotionally unavailable, the foundation of the relationship is undermined. The parent, once a secure base, becomes a figure of doubt or fear in the child's eyes. This shift, incongruent with the parent's actual behaviour, leads to a sharp decline in emotional closeness and may produce a pseudo-independence in the child that masks deep attachment confusion.

Shared Experiences

Alienated parents frequently grieve not only the absence of their child but also the irretrievable loss of shared experiences. Birthdays, school achievements, holidays, and everyday moments that form the fabric of a parent–child bond are missed. This absence of relational continuity creates a profound sense of dislocation and sadness. Parents often describe feeling like they are "erased" from their child's life narrative, reduced to an outsider in the most intimate and meaningful aspects of their child's development.

Persistent Difficulties

Even in cases where contact is later re-established, the psychological residue of alienation often lingers. Targeted parents may carry a persistent fear that alienation could recur, particularly if the underlying family dynamics or legal circumstances remain unresolved. This anticipatory anxiety can complicate reunification efforts, leading some parents to walk on emotional eggshells, reluctant to assert boundaries or express frustration, for fear of re-triggering rejection. As a result, even when physical proximity is restored, emotional intimacy may remain elusive.

The Questioning Child

In some cases, the child themselves may express confusion or guilt during reunification, particularly if they begin to question the narratives they were led to believe. This emotional ambivalence can be overwhelming for both parent and child, requiring sensitive therapeutic intervention to support the rebuilding of trust and mutual understanding. However, many targeted parents find that the scars of alienation, especially when prolonged or severe, leave lasting imprints on the relationship that may never fully heal.

Ultimately, the impact of PA on the parent–child relationship is not confined to a particular moment in time; it reshapes the trajectory of the bond, often leaving both parties with a legacy of pain, uncertainty, and longing. For targeted parents, the task of reconnection requires not only patience and emotional resilience but also recognition of the relational trauma that alienation has inflicted on both them and their child.

LEGAL AND FINANCIAL CONSEQUENCES

Significant legal and financial repercussions for the targeted parent often compound the experience of PA. These consequences extend beyond the psychological harm of relational loss, creating systemic pressures that deepen the sense of helplessness, destabilisation, and marginalisation that many parents already face. PA does not occur in a vacuum; it often unfolds within contentious legal processes that both reflect and reinforce the dynamics of alienation.

Ongoing Litigation and Custody Disputes

Targeted parents frequently find themselves embroiled in prolonged legal battles, often centred on child contact, custody arrangements, or allegations introduced by the alienating parent. These disputes can become cyclical, with repeated returns to court necessitated by non-compliance with orders, breaches of contact, or escalating accusations. Each legal encounter carries emotional, temporal, and psychological costs. The court system, while intended to arbitrate in the child's best interests, can inadvertently prolong the alienation if delays, inadequate assessments, or judicial misunderstanding allow alienating behaviours to persist unchallenged.

Financial Burden and Economic Instability

The legal processes surrounding PA often impose a substantial financial burden. Targeted parents may be required to fund legal representation, private psychological assessments, court-ordered interventions, and travel costs for supervised or limited contact. Many also report income loss due to missed workdays related to court hearings or child-related appointments. In extreme cases, parents are forced to deplete savings, sell property, or enter debt to sustain their involvement in legal proceedings, especially when litigation stretches over months or years.

Child Support Inequities and Economic Disempowerment

Financial pressures may be further intensified by complications surrounding child support. In some cases, targeted parents are required to continue paying substantial support despite being denied meaningful contact with their child, a situation many describe as both economically and ethically demoralising. Conversely, parents who are alienated but lack primary caregiving status may struggle to access financial resources needed to support litigation or therapeutic interventions, exacerbating inequalities in power and access to justice.

Professional and Reputational Fallout

PA may also carry consequences for the targeted parent's professional standing. False allegations, whether of abuse, neglect, or emotional instability, are sometimes circulated not only within the legal process but also among extended family, social networks, or workplaces. In high-conflict cases, alienating parents may engage in reputational smearing, spreading misinformation to undermine the targeted parent's credibility or social support. For those in public-facing or regulated professions, even unsubstantiated claims can damage career prospects, reduce employability, or lead to disciplinary scrutiny. The result is a compounding of losses: not only of parental identity and emotional security but also of financial stability and professional integrity.

Institutional Disempowerment and Systemic Injustice

A deep sense of systemic injustice often accompanies the combined legal and financial strain experienced by targeted parents. Many report feeling unheard, misrepresented, or even vilified by professionals within the family law and child protection systems. When legitimate concerns about alienation are misinterpreted as parental hostility or control, the very structures intended to safeguard family welfare can become instruments of further harm. This institutional disempowerment often compounds emotional trauma and may contribute to disengagement from the legal process altogether.

IMPACT ON WIDER FAMILY RELATIONSHIPS AND INTIMATE PARTNERSHIPS

The effects of PA reverberate far beyond the dyad of the targeted parent and the alienated child. PA disrupts the broader relational ecology in which the parent is embedded, affecting siblings, new partners, extended family, and future relationships. These collateral consequences often go unrecognised but carry significant emotional and psychological weight, further isolating the targeted parent and destabilising family systems.

Strain on Sibling Dynamics

When PA occurs in families with multiple children, it can fracture sibling relationships and create intense emotional divisions. Children who remain in contact with the targeted parent may feel caught between loyalties, torn between affection for a sibling and confusion about the rejection of a parent. In some cases, siblings adopt opposing positions, with one aligning with the alienating parent and another resisting. This can lead to conflict, guilt, and estrangement between siblings, compounding the grief experienced by the targeted parent, who not only loses access to one child but may witness the breakdown of sibling bonds as well.

Challenges for New Partners and Blended Families

New partners of targeted parents often find themselves drawn into the emotional fallout of PA. They may encounter resistance from the alienated child, who views them as an extension of the rejected parent, or they may be excluded from family routines and milestones altogether. In blended families, the tension can extend to stepchildren, who may struggle to understand the alienation or be indirectly impacted by the emotional strain in the household. The new partner may also feel helpless, frustrated, or unsupported, particularly if they witness the targeted parent's distress without knowing how to intervene constructively. Over time, this stress can destabilise the new relationship and erode the couple's emotional resilience. More on this in chapter 12.

Disruption of Extended Family Bonds

Extended family members, such as grandparents, aunts, uncles, and cousins, are often collateral victims of PA (see Chapter 12). Alienating parents may deliberately obstruct or sever these relationships, framing the extended family as complicit with the targeted parent or irrelevant to the child's wellbeing. For the alienated child, this results in the loss of rich intergenerational relationships, cultural continuity, and emotional support (as outlined in Chapter 10). For the targeted parents' family, it generates unresolved grief, feelings of exclusion, and, in some cases, long-term estrangement. These ruptures can also provoke conflict within the extended family itself, particularly if differing perspectives emerge regarding the alienation or how to respond to it.

Barriers to Future Intimacy and Trust

The experience of PA also often leaves a lasting psychological residue that impairs a targeted parent's capacity to engage in future intimate relationships. The trauma of unjust rejection, compounded by institutional invalidation and prolonged litigation, can generate chronic mistrust, emotional guardedness, or relational hypervigilance. Some targeted parents report difficulty forming new attachments, fearing that future partners may not understand or tolerate the complexities of their family history. Others may unconsciously carry expectations of loss or betrayal into new relationships, which can inhibit emotional closeness and limit the potential for healing.

LONG-TERM EFFECTS AND THE COMPLEX PATH TO HEALING

The effects of PA on targeted parents rarely end when court proceedings are finalised or when a child reaches adulthood. For many, the experience leaves behind psychological scars that alter not only their sense of self and relational capacity but also their long-term wellbeing and approach to parenting. Recovery is possible, but the journey is often lengthy, emotionally fraught, and shaped by ongoing uncertainty about whether reconciliation will ever occur.

Enduring Emotional and Psychological Consequences

Even after the active alienation subsides, through a change in custody, maturation of the child, or disengagement from the alienating parent, many targeted parents continue to experience unresolved grief, sadness, and emotional exhaustion. These feelings may manifest as chronic depression, anxiety, or complex trauma symptoms, particularly when the alienation has persisted for years without validation or effective intervention. Trust in others, including future partners, therapists, or even legal professionals, may be severely diminished, and targeted parents may struggle to re-establish a coherent sense of identity outside their parental role.

Parenting After Alienation

The alienation experience often casts a long shadow over how targeted parents approach future parenting relationships. Some become hypervigilant, fearing that any assertion of authority or boundary-setting could be interpreted as controlling or spark further rejection. Others may overcompensate, becoming overly permissive or emotionally enmeshed in an effort to avoid conflict or win affection. Both patterns can hinder the development of a healthy parent–child dynamic and may unintentionally reinforce the very anxieties the parent is trying to soothe. For parents who do reconnect with their child, renegotiating parenting roles can be both emotionally rewarding and extremely delicate, requiring patience, consistency, and support.

THE PROCESS OF HEALING

Healing from PA is not a linear process. It often requires targeted therapeutic support to help parents process the trauma, navigate the ambiguity of their loss, and rebuild their emotional resilience. Individual therapy can assist in addressing self-blame, shame, or symptoms of depression, while group support, particularly with other alienated parents, can provide much-needed validation and solidarity. In cases where the child is willing and the context permits, family therapy or reunification counselling may be helpful, though such interventions must be approached with care to avoid re-traumatisation or reinforcing coercive dynamics.

Healing also involves reclaiming a life beyond the alienation narrative. Many targeted parents report a gradual shift from identity solely as a parent to a more integrated sense of self that includes work, friendships, activism, and creative or spiritual pursuits. This broader identity reconstruction is often essential for long-term psychological recovery.

Reconciliation and Relational Repair

Although not always possible, reconciliation between targeted parents and their alienated children can occur, particularly as children reach adulthood and begin to question the narratives they have internalised. Such reunifications are often emotionally complex and may require long periods of incremental contact, emotional processing, and boundary setting. Rebuilding the relationship demands sustained emotional presence, humility, and a willingness to allow the child space to explore their own feelings without pressure. When successful, reconciliation can offer a profound opportunity for healing and closure, both for the parent and the child, but it is rarely straightforward and should be supported with therapeutic guidance wherever possible.

SUMMARY

This chapter has explored the profound psychological, emotional, and relational toll that parental alienation inflicts on targeted parents. While the focus of PA is often rightly on the child, it is essential to recognise that the alienated parent endures a form of invisible, ongoing trauma. This includes grief over a living child, feelings of helplessness, institutional invalidation, and a persistent sense of ambiguity and loss. Professionals working with alienated parents must understand that the emotional fallout mirrors the effects of coercive control, compounded by the lack of societal and legal recognition.

The mental health consequences are not only significant but can, in some cases, be life-threatening. Parents, especially fathers, are often pushed into psychological crisis, facing depression, anxiety, and, in extreme instances, suicidal ideation. Gendered expectations about emotional expression and systemic bias in family courts often mean that men, in particular, are left unsupported and misunderstood. These insights highlight the urgent need for clinicians and legal professionals to challenge assumptions about which parent is "at fault," and to consider how emotional distress might be a response to injustice, not evidence of unfitness.

Beyond the immediate rupture with their child, alienated parents face the erosion of meaningful relationships with other children, new partners, and extended family. The alienation often infects the wider family system, creating mistrust and disconnection. It can also impede future relational stability, as many parents emerge from the experience with deep psychological scars that affect their ability to trust, to parent confidently, or to reconnect without fear. Professionals must approach these cases systemically, recognising that alienation often has generational and familial consequences far beyond the presenting parent–child dyad.

Legal and financial consequences further compound the trauma of PA. Targeted parents may spend years entangled in costly and protracted litigation, often with minimal support or relief. False allegations, reputational damage, and punitive financial obligations can leave them economically depleted and socially stigmatised. For professionals in legal, social, or psychological roles, it is essential to appreciate how systemic failures can deepen alienation and push already vulnerable parents further into distress.

Recovery, though possible, is rarely straightforward. Healing from the experience of PA requires time, therapeutic support, and the rebuilding of identity outside of the parenting role. Some parents may achieve reconciliation with their child, particularly in adulthood, but this is emotionally complex and must be handled with sensitivity and patience. Practitioners must be cautious not to pathologise alienated parents but, rather, to validate their experience and provide trauma-informed interventions that acknowledge the deep relational wounds they carry.

Ultimately, professionals play a critical role in either reinforcing or challenging the dynamics of alienation. Whether in therapeutic settings, courtrooms, or community organisations, there is a responsibility to move beyond simplistic blame models and to develop nuanced understandings of how alienation operates, and how to support those caught in its grip.

BIBLIOGRAPHY

Balmer, S., Matthewson, M., & Haines, J. (2018). Parental alienation: Targeted parent perspective. *Australian Journal of Psychology*, *70*(1), 91–99. https://doi.org/10.1111/ajpy.12159

Bates, E. A., & Hine, B. A. (2023). "I was told when i could hold, talk with, or kiss our daughter": Exploring fathers' experiences of parental alienation within the context of intimate partner violence. *Partner Abuse*. https://doi.org/10.1891/PA-2022-0021

Hine, B. A., & Bates, E. A. (2023). "There is no part of my life that hasn't been destroyed": The impact of parental alienation and intimate partner violence on fathers. *Partner Abuse*. https://doi.org/10.1891/PA-2022-0058

Hine, B. A., & Hine, I. J. (2022). Fathers and intimate partner violence: An autoethnographic analysis of current literature on men's experiences of parental alienation In E. A. Bates & J. C. Taylor (Eds.), *Domestic violence against men and boys: Experiences of male victims of intimate partner violence*. Routledge.

Hine, B. A., & Roy, E. M. (2025). Supporting fathers experiencing family breakdown: Practitioner perspectives. *Social Sciences*, *14*(5), 232. https://doi.org/10.3390/socsci14050266

Hine, B. A., Roy, E. M., & Burhai, L. (2024). Father's experiences of family breakdown and domestic abuse. *Psychology of Men and Masculinities*, *26*, 265–274. https://doi.org/10.1037/men0000506

Hine, B. A., Roy, E. M., Huang, C. Y., & Bates, E. (2025a). Father's experiences of negotiating co-parenting arrangements and family court. *Social Sciences*, *14*(1), 29. https://doi.org/10.3390/socsci14010029

Hine, B. A., Roy, E. M., Huang, C. Y., & Bates, E. (2025b). Fathers' experiences of relationship breakdown including post-separation abuse and parental alienating behaviours. *Social Sciences*, *14*(1), 31. https://doi.org/10.3390/socsci14010031

Hine, B. A., Roy, E. M., Huang, C. Y., & Bates, E. (2025c). Impact of relationship breakdown, including abuse and negotiation of co-parenting arrangements, on fathers' mental health, help-seeking, and coping. *Social Sciences*, *14*(4), 232. https://doi.org/10.3390/socsci14040232

Lee-Maturana, S., Matthewson, M., & Dwan, C. (2020). Targeted parents surviving parental alienation: Consequences of the alienation and coping strategies. *Journal of Child and Family Studies*, *29*, 2268–2280. https://doi.org/10.1007/s10826-020-01725-1

Lee-Maturana, S., Matthewson, M., & Dwan, C. (2021). Understanding targeted parents' experience of parental alienation: A qualitative description from their own perspective. *The American Journal of Family Therapy*, *49*, 499–516. https://doi.org/10.1080/01926187.2020.1837035

Lee-Maturana, S., Matthewson, M., & Dwan, C. (2022). Ten key findings on targeted parents' expereince: Towards a broader definition of parental alienation. *Journal of Family Issues*, *43*, 2672–2700. https://doi.org/10.1177/0192513X211032664

Lee-Maturana, S., Matthewson, M., Dwan, C., & Norris, K. (2019). Characteristics and experiences of targeted parents of parental alienation from their own perspective: A systematic literature review. *Australian Journal of Psychology*, *71*, 83–91. https://doi.org/10.1111/ajpy.12226

Meland, E., Furuholmen, D., & Jahanlu, D. (2024). Parental alienation–a valid experience? *Scandinavian Journal of Public Health*, 52, 598–606. https://doi.org/10.1177/14034948231168978

Monk, L., & Bowen, E. (2021). Coercive control of women as mothers via strategic mother-child separation. *Journal of Gender-Based Violence*, 5, 23–42. https://doi.org/10.1332/239868020X15913793920878

Poustie, C., Matthewson, M., & Balmer, S. (2018). The forgotten parent: The targeted parent perspective of parental alienation. *Journal of Family Issues*, 39(12), 3298–3323. https://doi.org/10.1177/0192513X18777867

Sher, L. (2017). Parental alienation: The impact on men's mental health. *International Journal of Adolescent Medicine and Health*, 29. https://doi.org/10.1515/ijamh-2015-0083

Tavares, A., Crespo, C., & Ribeiro, M. T. (2020). Psychological adaptation and beliefs in targeted parents: A study in the context of parental alienation. *Journal of Child and Family Studies*, 29, 2281–2289. https://doi.org/10.1007/s10826-020-01742-0

Tavares, A., Crespo, C., & Ribeiro, M. T. (2021). What does it mean to be a targeted parent? Parents' experiences in the context of parental alienation. *Journal of Child and Family Studies*, 30, 1370–1380. https://doi.org/10.1007/s10826-021-01914-6

12

IMPACT ON THE WIDER FAMILY

PA is rarely confined to the parent–child relationship. Its effects reverberate outward, often destabilising the entire family system. Siblings, grandparents, extended relatives, and new partners of the targeted parent may all be drawn into the emotional fallout, experiencing loss, confusion, and relational strain as a result of the alienation. These individuals often find themselves cut off from the alienated child or navigating emotionally charged dynamics shaped by the conflict between parents. This chapter explores the multifaceted impact of PA on siblings, grandparents, wider family networks, and new or blended family structures, highlighting the emotional, relational, and systemic challenges they face in the shadow of alienation.

SIBLINGS

PA not only fractures the relationship between a child and a parent, but it also profoundly alters the relational terrain between siblings. Within families, each child exists in a triangulation formulation with their two parents. As a result, siblings may be positioned very differently within the same family narrative due to the dynamics within their own triangulation, with some becoming alienated and others maintaining bonds with the targeted parent. The divergent experiences that emerge from these triangulated structures can lead to confusion, competition, and emotional fragmentation among siblings.

DOI: 10.4324/9781003630944-16

In many cases, the alienation of one child generates ripple effects that deeply unsettle sibling dynamics. Children may experience conflicted loyalties, caught between their own relationship with a parent and their sibling's opposing stance. For some, the desire to stay connected to both parents can create inner turmoil, especially if the alienated sibling expresses hostility or moral certainty about rejecting the targeted parent. In this context, sibling relationships can become strained, with interactions marked by tension, silence, or attempts to recruit one another into alignment with a particular parent.

Emotional distress is therefore common. Siblings may feel helpless as they witness the breakdown of a relationship between their brother or sister and a parent they themselves still love. Others may carry guilt for maintaining a bond that their sibling has severed, or feel overwhelmed by the emotional complexity of trying to "stay neutral" in a situation that inherently demands allegiance. These dynamics often create an emotional burden that is difficult to articulate, especially for younger children or those without adequate adult support.

The alienation process can also fracture the sibling bond when roles are assigned within the family, either overtly or through subtle emotional cues. One sibling may be elevated as the "loyal" child, the emotional ally of the alienating parent, while another is framed as the outsider or potential betrayer. This may result in a "shining star" and a "scapegoat," with the alienating parent reinforcing these identities to maintain control and cohesion within their subsystem. These role divisions not only erode sibling solidarity but can also entrench long-term resentment, competition, and emotional estrangement.

Differential Impact

It is thus critical to recognise that PA is rarely a uniform experience across children within the same family. Different siblings may respond to the alienating parent's influence in varied ways, depending on factors such as age, temperament, prior attachment to each parent, or the timing and intensity of the alienation behaviours. One child may become fully alienated, another partially influenced, and a third may resist altogether. These variations can produce complex intra-family dynamics that exacerbate conflict and destabilise sibling relationships.

This asymmetry can heighten loyalty conflicts. A child who maintains a relationship with the targeted parent may feel pressure to conceal that bond from their alienated sibling, or risk being accused of betrayal. Conversely, the alienated sibling may experience distress or jealousy upon seeing their sibling receive affection from the parent they have rejected. These tensions often remain unspoken, yet they shape the emotional climate of the family, making genuine connection between siblings difficult to sustain.

The result is often a profound sense of fragmentation within the sibling unit. While some may attempt to mediate or bridge the divide, others may withdraw or internalise the conflict. Over time, these ruptures can harden into long-term estrangement, particularly if the alienation persists without intervention or if the family lacks access to therapeutic support.

In sum, PA can pit siblings against each other not only by shaping their views of each parent but by distorting how they see one another. The loss, then, is not only of parental connection but of sibling intimacy and shared belonging. Professionals working with alienated families must attend to these sibling dynamics explicitly, recognising the need to support each child's unique experience within the broader family conflict.

GRANDPARENTS

Grandparents, in particular, may find themselves unexpectedly cut off from their grandchildren as a result of the alienating parent's efforts to isolate the child from the targeted parent's familial network. Whether the alienation occurs after a meaningful bond has been established, or prevents a relationship from ever forming, the emotional and relational consequences for grandparents can be severe.

A primary impact is the loss of contact with grandchildren, often sudden and unexplained. Grandparents may be denied visits, communication, or even updates on the child's well-being. This rupture in the grandparent–grandchild relationship can provoke intense feelings of grief and mourning, akin to bereavement, but without closure. The loss is especially disorienting when the relationship was previously warm and active, and the disconnection occurs with no direct conflict or wrongdoing on the part of the grandparent.

The experience is often compounded by emotional distress, not only from the absence of the grandchild but also from witnessing their own adult child suffer through alienation. Many grandparents report feelings of helplessness, heartbreak, and deep frustration at their inability to protect or support either generation. These emotional burdens are intensified by the legal and social invisibility of grandparent alienation, which often leaves them with little recourse or support.

In many cases, PA introduces strain into broader family relationships. The alienating parent may work to control or fracture extended family dynamics, positioning some members as "allies" and others as "threats." Grandparents may find themselves forced to choose between supporting their adult child or maintaining access to the grandchild under increasingly restrictive or conditional terms. This dynamic can create long-term rifts within the family and undermine the support systems that many grandparents rely on in later life.

The reality of ageing often intensifies the emotional burden of grandparent alienation. For many grandparents, the experience of being cut off from their grandchildren comes at a stage of life when physical health may already be in decline, and psychological resilience is often reduced. The stress associated with prolonged alienation can exacerbate existing health conditions, such as cardiovascular issues, autoimmune problems, or insomnia, and is frequently accompanied by symptoms of chronic grief, depression, and anxiety. Many express a painful sense that they are "running out of time," not only to witness their grandchildren grow up, but to pass on family stories, cultural traditions, and personal legacies. This awareness can lead to feelings of despair and urgency, compounding the emotional strain and making the loss feel even more permanent. For some, this sense of irretrievable time lost becomes one of the most devastating aspects of the experience. There may also be financial implications, especially when grandparents contribute to the legal costs of their alienated adult child. These contributions, often made out of desperation to help preserve the family bond, can place significant strain on the financial well-being of older adults, many of whom are on fixed incomes.

Differential Impact on Grandparents

Just as the experience of PA varies among siblings, it also affects grandparents in diverse and complex ways. While some have their established relationships with grandchildren abruptly severed, others are denied the opportunity to develop a relationship from the outset. These two scenarios present distinct, but equally painful, forms of alienation.

For grandparents who had a pre-existing relationship with their grandchildren, the sudden disconnection can be emotionally devastating. They often describe feelings of betrayal, confusion, and deep sorrow, particularly when the alienation occurs without explanation or justification. The loss of shared routines, holidays, and emotional intimacy can feel akin to losing the grandchild entirely, despite their continued physical presence in the world.

By contrast, grandparents who have never met their grandchildren must contend with the pain of a relationship that was never allowed to begin. This anticipatory grief, mourning a connection they hoped for but were denied, can be equally profound. These individuals often express a sense of being robbed of a core life experience, particularly as grandparenthood is often anticipated as a vital stage of later life. This can lead to enduring feelings of loss, loneliness, and alienation from the family legacy.

In both cases, alienated grandparents frequently encounter barriers to help-seeking, including disbelief from professionals, lack of legal standing, and societal minimisation of their role. While some find validation and support through counselling or peer groups, others report feeling misunderstood or dismissed by practitioners unfamiliar with the dynamics of PA.

Ultimately, the impact of PA on grandparents underscores the wide-reaching consequences of relational disruption within the family system. Professionals working in mental health, elder care, and family services must be equipped to recognise the legitimacy of grandparent grief, and to offer informed, empathetic support that validates their experiences and helps mitigate isolation.

The Role of Grandparents on the Alienating Parent's Side

While much attention is rightly given to the experience of grandparents connected to the targeted parent, the role of the alienating parent's own parents is equally complex and often overlooked. Grandparents on the alienating side of the family may either reinforce the alienation, intentionally or passively, or find themselves deeply conflicted by their child's behaviour and unsure how to respond.

In some cases, grandparents may become active participants in the alienation process, supporting their adult child's narrative and reinforcing the child's rejection of the targeted parent. This can occur for a variety of reasons: loyalty to their child, unresolved historical conflict with the targeted parent, or a sincere, but misinformed, belief that they are protecting the grandchild. These grandparents may speak negatively about the targeted parent, limit the child's access to alternative perspectives, or reward signs of loyalty to the alienating parent. When this occurs, the intergenerational transmission of alienation is further entrenched, embedding family division more deeply across generations.

Conversely, some grandparents on the alienating side may feel deeply distressed by the role their child is playing in the estrangement. They may disagree with the alienating behaviours, but feel powerless to intervene, either for fear of damaging their own access to the grandchild or out of concern for provoking further conflict. These grandparents may attempt to act as mediators or quietly maintain a neutral stance, but often find themselves marginalised or silenced if their views conflict with the alienating parent's agenda. The emotional toll of witnessing their grandchild being used as a tool of coercion or manipulation can be significant, particularly when paired with guilt about their own child's involvement in the process.

In both scenarios, the grandparents on the alienating side of the family are navigating a morally and emotionally fraught landscape. Some may eventually experience estrangement themselves if they attempt to challenge the alienation, while others remain enmeshed in a system that discourages dissent. For professionals, it is important not to assume a monolithic stance among extended family members but to assess each individual's role, beliefs, and capacity to influence or disrupt the alienation dynamic. With appropriate support and psychoeducation, some of these grandparents may become valuable allies in restoring balance and supporting the child's access to both sides of their family.

NEW PARTNERS AND BLENDED FAMILIES

PA often spills into the lives of new partners and blended families, introducing emotional complexity, relational strain, and uncertainty into already delicate dynamics. These individuals are frequently drawn into a high-conflict family environment that predates their involvement. Yet, they may bear the emotional and relational consequences without having full insight into, or control over, the situation. For new partners, whether romantically involved with the targeted parent or forming part of a broader blended household, the effects of PA can be distressing and disorienting.

A common challenge faced by new partners is the difficulty in building relationships with the child who has been alienated. The child, already caught in a loyalty conflict and influenced by the alienating parent's narrative, may view the new partner with suspicion, resistance, or outright hostility. Efforts to connect are often met with emotional withdrawal or rejection, leaving the new partner feeling excluded, unwanted, or unsure of how to engage appropriately. This can be especially painful when the new partner is actively trying to provide support or offer a stable family environment.

In addition to relationship difficulties with the child, new partners often experience significant emotional distress as they witness the targeted parent's suffering and the breakdown of family connections. The emotional labour of supporting a partner through alienation, while navigating their own place in a conflicted family system, can lead to feelings of helplessness, anxiety, or burnout. This distress is often compounded by the lack of recognition or support available to new partners, whose experiences are rarely centralised in professional or legal responses to PA.

The relationship between the new partner and the alienating parent can also be a source of conflict. Alienating parents may perceive new partners as intruders, competitors, or destabilising forces, and may actively attempt to undermine their involvement. This could include disparaging the new partner in front of the child, refusing to acknowledge their role in the child's life, or using legal and procedural tactics to disrupt family routines. These actions not only damage the potential for constructive co-parenting but also place the new partner in a precarious position, emotionally invested but excluded from meaningful influence.

Blended families as a whole can also be adversely affected. When a new partner has children of their own, the tensions caused by PA may ripple through the household, straining sibling-like relationships and destabilising routines. Children from previous relationships may feel confused or upset by the conflict they observe, and the emotional energy required to manage the alienation may reduce the attention available for other relationships within the home. Over time, these pressures can threaten the cohesion and stability of the blended family, particularly if they are not addressed with open communication, professional support, and realistic expectations.

Professionals supporting families experiencing PA should be mindful of the emotional burden placed on new partners and blended families. Their perspectives are often overlooked, yet they play a critical role in the emotional environment of the targeted parent and in the broader efforts to maintain relational stability for the child. Validating their experiences, clarifying roles and boundaries, and equipping them with tools to manage high-conflict dynamics can all contribute to better outcomes for families navigating the complexities of parental alienation.

Financial Strain

One of the most under-recognised, yet profoundly impactful, aspects of PA is the financial strain it places on new partners and blended families. While emotional and relational challenges are more commonly acknowledged, the economic toll of living within a high-conflict post-separation dynamic can significantly destabilise new households. This issue warrants special focus, as financial stress often amplifies pre-existing emotional tensions and can jeopardise the long-term sustainability of blended family relationships.

Legal expenses represent one of the most immediate and burdensome financial pressures. As targeted parents often face extended court proceedings to maintain or regain contact with their children, new partners may become indirectly responsible for covering part of these costs, whether through shared resources, lost income, or by deferring their own financial priorities. This financial entanglement can create resentment, especially if the legal battle becomes prolonged or adversarial, and may strain the trust and security within the new partnership.

In addition to legal fees, therapy and counselling costs can accrue as the family attempts to cope with the emotional fallout of PA. Whether directed towards the targeted parent, the alienated child, or the new partner themselves, therapeutic support is often necessary, but rarely inexpensive. These expenses may not be budgeted for and can add further strain to a household already under pressure from the emotional consequences of alienation.

There are also hidden financial costs that arise from the time and emotional labour required to navigate life alongside PA. New partners often invest significant time supporting their partner through distress, advocating for the child, or managing crisis points that arise from contact disputes or legal confrontations. This emotional caregiving can come at the expense of their own career progression, paid work availability, or educational pursuits, ultimately reducing household income and opportunities.

For blended families trying to establish a sense of normalcy, these financial burdens can destabilise the very foundation they are trying to build. They may also limit the family's ability to invest in positive shared experiences, such as holidays, outings, or extracurricular activities, that could otherwise help strengthen bonds and provide much-needed emotional respite.

Professionals working with alienated families should take care not to overlook the economic dimensions of PA's impact. Addressing financial stress openly, validating the sacrifices being made by new partners, and referring families to appropriate legal and financial resources can all help to mitigate the long-term strain and preserve the well-being of blended family units navigating the challenges of alienation.

Risk of Contributing to Alienation: The Role of New Partners on Both Sides

While new partners can offer crucial emotional support and stability in families affected by PA, their involvement also carries risk, particularly when their actions or attitudes, even if well intentioned, contribute to escalating or reinforcing alienation. This dynamic is not exclusive to the new partners of targeted parents. New partners of alienating parents can also play a significant role in either amplifying or mitigating the alienation process, often without full awareness of the underlying dynamics or long-term implications for the child.

New Partners of Targeted Parents

For new partners of targeted parents, the emotional toll of witnessing unjust rejection or institutional invalidation can evoke strong feelings of anger, frustration, and helplessness. In some cases, this may lead to negative expressions about the alienating parent, spoken in the child's presence or indirectly conveyed through body language, tone, or emotional withdrawal. Although these responses are understandable, they risk entrenching the child further into the loyalty conflict, reinforcing the narrative that they must choose between households or identities.

Moreover, in the effort to support their partner and bond with the child, some new partners may inadvertently engage in behaviours that mirror alienation dynamics. For example, they may consciously or unconsciously frame themselves as a superior caregiver, dismiss the child's relationship with the other parent, or encourage emotional dependency as a way to foster closeness. This can further confuse the child, intensify their internal conflict, and contribute to a dynamic in which both parents, and their respective households, become adversarial in the child's mind.

New Partners of Alienating Parents

New partners who join families where alienation is already underway may also be drawn into the process, sometimes co-opted into reinforcing the alienating narrative. In seeking to integrate themselves into the existing family structure, or gain the approval of the alienating parent, they may accept negative portrayals of the targeted parent without question. In more concerning cases, they may become active participants in the alienation by repeating false narratives, limiting contact opportunities, or discouraging the child from expressing affection towards the targeted parent.

However, not all new partners of alienating parents are complicit. Some find themselves deeply conflicted, recognising the damage being caused but unsure how to intervene without jeopardising their own relationship. These individuals may experience moral discomfort, or feel silenced within a dynamic where questioning the dominant narrative is discouraged or punished. For these partners, opportunities for reflection and education can be crucial in breaking the cycle of alienation.

Given the decisive role that new partners can play on both sides of an alienated family system, professional guidance is essential. New partners often lack the necessary context or training to understand fully the impact of their actions, and may greatly benefit from psychoeducation, counselling, or family therapy. Encouraging new partners to maintain a reflective stance, avoiding blame, resisting polarised thinking, and prioritising the child's emotional needs can help to reduce the risk of further alienation and foster a healthier family climate.

SUMMARY

Parental alienation rarely confines its damage to the relationship between a parent and child; rather, it fractures the entire family ecosystem. Siblings may be positioned differently within triangulated dynamics, one cast as the "loyal" child and another as the "scapegoat," resulting in disrupted sibling bonds, unspoken loyalty conflicts, and long-term estrangement. Grandparents, too, suffer deeply, whether through the abrupt loss of once-close relationships or the devastation of never meeting their grandchildren. The ageing process can amplify this grief, with many expressing a desperate sense of "running out of time," compounded by health deterioration, financial strain, and social invisibility. Notably, even grandparents on the alienating parent's side face complex emotional terrain; some inadvertently reinforce the alienation, while others are marginalised for dissenting from it.

New partners and blended families face unique emotional, relational, and financial stressors, often absorbing the emotional fallout of a conflict they did not initiate. These partners may struggle to build relationships with alienated children, endure attacks from the alienating parent, or risk unintentionally deepening the divide. Financial burdens, from legal fees to therapeutic support, can strain household stability and erode emotional resilience. Crucially, both new partners of targeted and alienating parents may unknowingly reinforce the alienation if not adequately informed or supported. As such, professionals must approach extended family members and blended units as integral, not peripheral, to the PA dynamic.

Professionals working with alienated families should adopt a systemic lens, recognising that each member, including siblings, grandparents, and new partners, may be grappling with unique forms of loss, confusion, and moral distress. Validating these experiences, offering psychoeducation, and tailoring interventions to address the whole family system, not just the parent–child dyad, are essential steps in mitigating harm and promoting healing across generations.

BIBLIOGRAPHY

Avieli, H., & Levy, I. (2023). "I feel erased:" A qualitative analysis of grandparent experiences of parental alienation. *Family Relations, 72*, 976–992. https://doi.org/10.1111/fare.12704

Bounds, O., & Matthewson, M. (2023). Parental alienating behaviours experienced by alienated grandparents. *Journal of Family Issues, 44*, 3250–3272. https://doi.org/10.1177/0192513X221126753

Degges-White, S., Hermann-Turner, K., Kepic, M., Randolph, A., & Killam, W. (2024). Grandparent alienation: A mixed method exploration of life satisfaction and help-seeking experiences of grandparents alienated from their grandchildren. *The Family Journal*. https://doi.org/10.1177/10664807241282432

Golly, C. H. (2016). Pruning the family tree: The plight of grandparents who are alienated from their grandchildren. *The Journal of Aging and Social Change, 7*, 21.

Kruk, E., & Varavei, H. (2025). The lived experiences of grandparents who have never seen their grandchildren: A new perspective on grandparent alienation. *Ageing International, 50*, 1–28. https://doi.org/10.1007/s12126-025-09601-3

Marsden, J. (2025). *The effects of parental alienation on sibling relationships and the sibling subsystem: A grounded theory study*. Manuscript in Preparation.

PART 4

WHAT CAN WE DO ABOUT IT?

13

CHALLENGING PARENTAL ALIENATION EARLY

PA is best addressed before it fully develops, through proactive, systemic strategies aimed at prevention and early intervention. These include strengthening parent–child relationships, supporting positive co-parenting following separation, and fostering cultural discourses that resist adversarial conceptions of post-separation parenting.

BUILDING AND MAINTAINING HEALTHY PARENT–CHILD RELATIONSHIPS

Strong, emotionally secure relationships between children and their parents act as a protective buffer against the effects of alienating behaviours. Even when separation occurs, such bonds can offer resistance to the psychological manipulations that characterise PA. Strategies that help establish and sustain healthy relationships include:

- *Prioritising relational presence:* Intentional time spent with children in meaningful activities strengthens emotional bonds and generates shared narratives that are more resistant to external interference.
- *Facilitating open communication:* Children should feel safe discussing their experiences, including ambivalent or complex feelings about each parent. Avoiding judgement, modelling active listening, and validating

DOI: 10.4324/9781003630944-18

emotions can create the kind of relational safety that alienation disrupts.

- *Demonstrating emotional availability:* Being consistently attuned to a child's emotional needs, especially during and after separation, fosters a secure base and mitigates the vulnerability to emotional manipulation.
- *Reinforcing autonomy and secure attachment:* Healthy parent–child dynamics involve boundaries that promote both connection and individuality. This supports the development of a stable self-concept, reducing the likelihood that children will internalise distorted narratives about one parent.
- *Remaining child-centred:* Taking an interest in the child's world – their friends, fears, goals, and identity – reinforces the legitimacy and value of the parent–child bond, which is central to resilience against alienation.

PROMOTING HEALTHY CO-PARENTING POST-SEPARATION

PA rarely occurs in isolation; it is typically embedded in a broader ecology of conflict, attachment disruption, and post-separation power struggles. The quality of co-parenting post-separation is among the most significant factors influencing whether alienation occurs. Key strategies include:

- *Constructive communication and conflict management:* Co-parents who can separate their relationship dynamics from their parenting responsibilities are more likely to maintain a cooperative stance, reducing the conditions under which alienation thrives.
- *Keeping the child's needs paramount:* Effective co-parenting means prioritising the child's psychological safety over adult grievances. This includes fostering the child's right to a full relationship with both parents, barring legitimate risk.
- *Utilising structured supports:* Mediation, collaborative divorce processes, and parenting coordination services can de-escalate conflict and reinforce shared responsibilities. These interventions are especially important in high-conflict cases.
- *Establishing detailed parenting plans:* Clear, enforceable parenting plans that include decision-making roles, routines, and contingencies help reduce ambiguity – a condition that often fuels alienating dynamics.
- *Promoting mutual affirmation:* A critical protective factor is each parent actively supporting the child's relationship with the other parent. This includes avoiding negative talk, resisting triangulation, and modelling respect even in the face of unresolved conflict.
- *Accessing education and guidance:* Programmes designed to teach conflict resolution, attachment-aware parenting, and post-separation dynamics can equip parents with skills that directly mitigate the risk of PA.

SOCIETAL DISCOURSES AND THE ROLE OF CULTURE IN PREVENTING PA

Beyond families, broader societal narratives about separation, parenting, and custody arrangements shape how alienation is understood and either challenged or enabled.

- *Challenging adversarial discourses:* Popular and legal narratives often frame separation as a zero-sum conflict, reinforcing loyalty traps and power contests. A culture that frames parenting as a collaborative, lifelong responsibility, regardless of the status of the adult relationship, can provide protective scaffolding.
- *Addressing gendered assumptions:* As highlighted in earlier chapters, societal assumptions about parental roles can obscure the reality of PA. Mothers and fathers alike can be perpetrators or victims of alienating behaviours. Challenging gendered stereotypes in legal, clinical, and cultural settings is essential.
- *Normalising support-seeking:* Societies must destigmatise the emotional fallout of separation and encourage parents to seek professional help early. Alienation often develops in contexts where psychological distress is left unaddressed.
- *Promoting child rights frameworks:* Viewing children as autonomous individuals with rights, rather than as extensions of one parent, can shift discourses away from parental entitlement and towards relational responsibility.
- *Educating communities:* Schools, religious institutions, and local services all play a role in identifying early signs of PA and supporting affected families. Public awareness campaigns can also help reduce stigma and misinformation.

THE BENEFITS OF 50:50 SHARED CARE IN MITIGATING PARENTAL ALIENATION

The presumption of 50:50 shared care following separation is gaining traction in some jurisdictions, reflecting a growing recognition of the value of continued, meaningful relationships with both parents after family breakdown. While this model is not universally appropriate (as explored in the following section), when implemented thoughtfully, it offers a number of protective benefits, particularly in mitigating the emergence of alienating dynamics and reinforcing the child's right to relational continuity.

Promoting Secure Attachment Across Households

From an attachment perspective, regular and meaningful engagement with both parents helps children maintain secure internal working models of care, even amidst family restructuring. Consistent exposure to both parents can preserve the attachment bonds that serve as emotional anchors for children, reducing anxiety, confusion, and vulnerability to manipulation by one parent against the other. In the absence of such continuity, children may be more susceptible to developing distorted loyalties or internalising a narrative of abandonment or rejection.

Reducing Power Asymmetries That Enable Alienation

A consistent finding in the literature on parental alienation is that it often arises in contexts of asymmetrical power post-separation, typically when one parent has disproportionate control over the child's time, narratives, or emotional access. Shared care reduces the opportunity for one parent to become the "gatekeeper" of the child's perceptions, experiences, and relational history. By maintaining both parents in active roles, shared care can act as a structural deterrent to alienating behaviours.

Normalising Both Parents' Ongoing Role

Shared care arrangements send a strong message to the child that both parents remain central to their life, regardless of the breakdown of the adult relationship. This reinforces the idea that parental love and involvement are enduring, stable, and non-conditional, countering the polarised narratives that often accompany alienation. It also normalises the coexistence of two nurturing figures in the child's emotional landscape, fostering psychological flexibility and security.

Encouraging Cooperative Co-Parenting

While high-conflict cases may initially resist shared parenting frameworks, structured 50:50 arrangements can, paradoxically, reduce long-term conflict by clarifying roles, reducing feelings of injustice, and discouraging the use of the child as leverage. Equal parenting time can decrease competition and reframe the parental relationship as one of mutual responsibility rather than contested authority. Moreover, courts and mediators have increasingly recognised that when both parents feel heard, seen, and engaged, the incentive to alienate often diminishes.

Enhancing Relational Diversity and Stability for the Child

Each parent brings a unique set of strengths, routines, cultural practices, extended family relationships, and parenting styles. Maintaining access to both these worlds expands the child's developmental and social ecology. This breadth of experience enriches their identity and contributes to a more robust emotional foundation, particularly important in times of familial upheaval.

Safeguarding Against Narrative Distortion

Children in sole-custody arrangements are more likely to become reliant on the dominant parent's account of the separation, the other parent's character, and their own early experiences. In contrast, regular engagement with both parents allows children to draw upon direct relational experience rather than second-hand narratives. This is especially critical in preventing the cognitive and emotional distortions that often characterise alienation, such as splitting, idealisation of one parent, and the demonisation of the other.

Empirical Support for Better Outcomes

Evidence from multiple jurisdictions suggests that children in shared care arrangements tend to exhibit better outcomes across a range of domains, including mental health, academic performance, and social functioning, than those in sole-custody situations, particularly when parental conflict is not extreme. These findings reinforce the principle that, where safe and feasible, children benefit from the continued presence and involvement of both parents.

However, it is important to note that while shared care arrangements can promote balanced parenting and reduce opportunities for alienating behaviours, they are not a universal solution. The presumption of equal time must be weighed against the specific needs and risks present in each case. Important considerations include:

- The age and developmental needs of the child
- The geographical and logistical feasibility of shared care
- The level and type of parental conflict
- Any history of abuse, neglect, or coercive control

A blanket approach to 50:50 care may inadvertently expose children to risk or entrench control dynamics. However, where safely possible, shared parenting reinforces the child's attachment to both parents and can disrupt the power asymmetries that often underlie PA.

RECOGNISING AND RESPONDING TO EARLY SIGNS OF PA

Early signs of PA often go unnoticed or are misattributed to ordinary post-separation adjustment. However, timely recognition can prevent the entrenchment of alienating behaviours. Indicators may include:

- Disproportionate fear, hostility, or rejection towards one parent without a clear, legitimate cause
- Use of adult-like or scripted language to describe the targeted parent
- Sudden cessation of affectionate behaviours
- Idealisation of one parent and demonisation of the other

- Anxiety, distress, or physical symptoms (e.g., nausea) before contact with the targeted parent

When such signs are observed, early steps include:

- *Open dialogue and validation:* Allowing children to express their experiences without interrogation or invalidation is vital.
- *Therapeutic engagement:* Specialist therapists can assess whether the child's rejection is justified (estrangement) or manipulated (alienation), guiding appropriate responses.
- *Cross-professional collaboration:* Schools, healthcare providers, and legal professionals must share relevant insights and coordinate responses in suspected PA cases.
- *Education and upskilling:* Parents and professionals alike should understand the distinction between PA and other contact issues (estrangement, loyalty conflicts, gatekeeping), as explored in Chapter 2.

THE ROLE OF EXTENDED FAMILY AND COMMUNITY NETWORKS

Extended family members and community actors can serve as buffers or enablers of PA. They may:

- *Provide a stabilising presence:* Maintaining connection with grandparents, cousins, and non-residential relatives affirms the child's place in a wider relational ecosystem.
- *Reinforce balanced narratives:* Trusted adults can offer non-polarised stories about both parents, countering distorted or binary messaging.
- *Act as mediators:* In high-conflict scenarios, third parties can support communication or clarify misperceptions.
- *Spot manipulation early:* Observers outside the immediate parental dyad may be the first to notice emerging patterns of alienation.

IMPLEMENTING EARLY INTERVENTION STRATEGIES

Beyond awareness, early intervention must be proactive, collaborative, and tailored to the dynamics of each case. Key approaches include:

- *Family therapy:* Can address underlying relational fractures, clarify misperceptions, and rebuild trust, though only when both parents engage constructively.
- *Individual therapy for children and parents:* Can help clarify the child's authentic feelings, support emotional regulation, and reduce loyalty conflicts.
- *Parent coordination services:* These structured interventions are crucial in managing high-conflict parenting and ensuring accountability to agreed arrangements.

- *Legal safeguards:* Protective orders, monitored contact, or modifications to parenting plans may be necessary where one parent persistently undermines the child's relationship with the other.

SUMMARY

Preventing and intervening early in cases of parental alienation is not simply a matter of better parenting. It is a systemic task that requires relational, psychological, legal, and cultural insight. By strengthening healthy attachments, fostering respectful co-parenting, recognising early signs of alienation, and challenging adversarial discourses around separation, we can better protect children from the lasting harms of PA and promote resilience across family systems. The next chapter provides practical advice to help implement these points for everyone involved.

BIBLIOGRAPHY

Bastaits, K., & Pasteels, I. (2019). Is joint physical custody in the best interests of the child? Parent–child relationships and custodial arrangements. *Journal of Social and Personal Relationships*, 36(11–12), 3752–3772. https://doi.org/10.1177/026540751983807

Bergström, M., Fransson, E., Fabian, H., Hjern, A., Sarkadi, A., & Salari, R. (2018). Preschool children living in joint physical custody arrangements show less psychological symptoms than those living mostly or only with one parent. *Acta Paediatrica*, 107(2), 294–300. https://doi.org/10.1111/apa.14004

Braver, S. L., & Lamb, M. E. (2018). Shared parenting after parental separation: The views of 12 experts. *Journal of Divorce & Remarriage*, 59(5), 372–387. https://doi.org/10.1080/10502556.2018.1454195

Mahrer, N. E., O'hara, K. L., Sandler, I. N., & Wolchik, S. A. (2018). Does shared parenting help or hurt children in high-conflict divorced families? *Journal of Divorce & Remarriage*, 59(4), 324–347. https://doi.org/10.1080/10502556.2018.1454200

Nielsen, L. (2011). Shared parenting after divorce: A review of shared residential parenting research. *Journal of Divorce & Remarriage*, 52(8), 586–609. https://doi.org/10.1080/10502556.2011.619913

Nielsen, L. (2018a). Joint versus sole physical custody: Children's outcomes independent of parent–child relationships, income, and conflict in 60 studies. *Journal of Divorce & Remarriage*, 59(4), 247–281. https://doi.org/10.1080/10502556.2018.1454204

Nielsen, L. (2018b). Joint versus sole physical custody: Outcomes for children independent of family income or parental conflict. *Journal of Child Custody*, 15(1), 35–54. https://doi.org/10.1080/15379418.2017.1422414

Ortega-Gaspar, M., Moreno-Mínguez, A., & López-Narbona, A. (2022). Impact of joint physical custody and best interest of the child: Reflections from a critical review of empirical studies. *Journal of Divorce & Remarriage*, 63(2), 101–119. https://doi.org/10.1080/10502556.2021.1993014

Steinbach, A. (2019). Children's and parents' well-being in joint physical custody: A literature review. *Family Process*, 58(2), 353–369. https://doi.org/10.1111/famp.12372

Steinbach, A., Augustijn, L., & Corkadi, G. (2021). Joint physical custody and adolescents' life satisfaction in 37 North American and European countries. *Family Process*, 60(1), 145–158. https://doi.org/10.1111/famp.12536

14

ADVICE ON EARLY INTERVENTION

In the previous chapter, we explored why early intervention is critical to mitigating the development and entrenchment of PA. We examined how fostering secure parent–child relationships, promoting healthy co-parenting, and reshaping adversarial cultural discourses can serve as protective factors against alienation. Building on this foundation, the current chapter offers practical guidance tailored to three key audiences: (1) parents navigating the early stages of separation or exposure to alienating behaviours, (2) children and young people experiencing the emotional and relational disruptions of PA, and (3) professionals, particularly those in legal, clinical, and educational roles, tasked with identifying, supporting, and intervening in cases of early-stage alienation. Each section provides evidence-informed strategies designed to prevent the escalation of alienation, promote relational repair, and safeguard the psychological wellbeing of affected family members.

ADVICE FOR PARENTS EXPERIENCING SEPARATION AND EARLY ALIENATION

Separation and divorce are emotionally complex events that can disrupt family dynamics and place significant strain on parent–child relationships. In this context, it is vital that parents proactively adopt strategies that foster resilience, preserve attachment bonds, and mitigate the risk of early alienating behaviours taking root. The following guidance is designed for parents at

DOI: 10.4324/9781003630944-19

the onset of separation, as well as those beginning to recognise subtle indications of relational disruption, triangulation, or loyalty conflicts. Many of these points can also be implemented by parents who are still in relationships and experiencing these behaviours.

Maintain a Child-Centred Focus

During separation, it is essential to centre the child's psychological safety and relational continuity above all else. Parents should always ask, "What does my child need to feel emotionally safe and secure?" Rather than viewing parenting time as a commodity to be won or lost, parents are encouraged to adopt the framework of relational stewardship, working to preserve the child's right to love and be loved by both parents, regardless of adult grievances.

Avoid Negative Talk and Emotional Triangulation

One of the earliest markers of potential alienation is the subtle undermining of the other parent through criticism, sarcasm, or emotional leakage. Even offhand remarks made in the child's hearing can create loyalty conflicts. Parents should:

- Refrain from speaking negatively about the other parent, even when the relationship is strained.
- Avoid making the child a confidant in adult matters, including legal proceedings or financial concerns.
- Respect the child's freedom to form their own relationship with the other parent, free from coercion or manipulation.

Establish Structured, Predictable Contact

Children experiencing family breakdown benefit from structure, routine, and consistency. Establishing clear parenting schedules with mutual agreement reinforces stability and reduces opportunities for one parent to control access or narratives. Where possible:

- Implement a detailed parenting plan early, including holidays, handovers, and communication protocols.
- Use written agreements or mediation services to ensure clarity and accountability, especially if informal arrangements become contested.

Encourage Open Dialogue and Emotional Expression

Children may internalise confusion or distress when family dynamics shift. Parents can provide a buffer against alienation by actively encouraging the child to express feelings without fear of reprisal or allegiance-testing. This includes:

- Validating the child's emotions, even when they are difficult to hear.
- Reassuring the child that it is acceptable to love both parents.
- Modelling reflective listening and non-defensive responses.

Respond Early to Signs of Distancing or Rejection

When a child begins showing signs of alignment with one parent and withdrawal from the other, it is crucial to intervene early with sensitivity and curiosity, not confrontation. Early signs may include:

- Sudden or uncharacteristic resistance to spending time with one parent.
- Adoption of language or narratives that mirror the aligned parent.
- Anxious or avoidant behaviour around transitions between households.

Where these signs emerge, parents are advised to seek professional input, ideally from practitioners trained in attachment, family systems, or parental alienation dynamics. Importantly, interventions at this stage are typically more effective and less invasive than those required in entrenched cases.

Embrace a Co-Parenting Mindset, Even Without Reciprocity

While ideal co-parenting requires mutual effort, one parent adopting a collaborative, non-retaliatory stance can still exert a protective effect on the child. This includes:

- Providing consistent emotional availability, even if the child is ambivalent or distant.
- Maintaining respectful communication with the other parent, even when it is not reciprocated.
- Documenting concerns factually and constructively without fuelling conflict or drawing the child into disputes.

Engage with Professional and Peer Support

Early-stage alienation often leaves parents feeling isolated, confused, or gaslit. Seeking support is not a sign of weakness but a proactive step towards resilience. Parents are encouraged to:

- Consult professionals with specific expertise in high-conflict family dynamics and alienation.

- Join support networks or groups for separating parents that emphasise child-centred approaches.
- Avoid forums or communities that reinforce adversarial thinking or promote entrenched hostility.

Avoid Retaliation or Mirroring of Alienating Behaviours

It is natural to feel angry, betrayed, or desperate when beginning to suspect alienating dynamics. However, mirroring these behaviours, through gatekeeping, counter-narratives, or rigid control, risks exacerbating the conflict and further destabilising the child. Instead, parents should:

- Anchor responses in the child's long-term wellbeing, not short-term emotional vindication.
- Maintain relational consistency and reliability, providing the child with an emotionally safe alternative to polarisation.
- Trust that even when the child is temporarily influenced, consistent care leaves a lasting impression.

Stay Grounded and Remain a Steady Presence

Perhaps the most powerful gift a parent can offer a child during and after separation is a consistent, calm presence. Even in the face of intense adversity, false allegations, rejection, or overt hostility, it is critical to maintain emotional composure and avoid being drawn into reactive patterns, no matter how hard this is to do. Children are acutely sensitive to emotional atmospheres, and while they may not always show it, they are deeply affected by the steadiness or volatility of parental behaviour. Remaining grounded means:

- Responding rather than reacting to provocations or manipulation.
- Protecting the child from adult conflict, regardless of your own pain or frustration.
- Demonstrating that your love is unconditional and not contingent upon the child's behaviour or expressed loyalty.

When a child witnesses one parent remaining calm, loving, and present, even when being rejected or misrepresented, it creates a powerful counter-narrative to alienation. Over time, such consistency can help the child reconcile conflicting emotions, challenge distorted beliefs, and feel safe to reconnect. This kind of quiet resilience, though often unseen in the moment, lays the groundwork for future healing and relational restoration.

BUT – Know Your Ex-Partner's Profile – and Adjust Expectations Accordingly

The success of many early interventions depends not only on what you do as a parent but also on *who* you are parenting alongside. While some ex-partners may behave in alienating ways due to temporary distress or emotional wounding, others may operate from more entrenched, pathological patterns that are resistant to change. Understanding the difference is crucial.

When the alienating behaviours arise from situational pain or unresolved conflict, many of the strategies in this section, empathy, calm consistency, respectful boundaries, and open communication, can help shift the dynamic. These parents, though hurting, may still respond to child-centred approaches or professional mediation over time.

However, if your ex-partner is exhibiting persistent, controlling, or psychologically manipulative behaviour, particularly when aligned with traits such as narcissism, entitlement, or lack of empathy, then you may be dealing with a more pathological dynamic. In these cases, expecting reciprocity, fairness, or shared concern for the child's best interests may be unrealistic and emotionally costly.

If you suspect this may be the case, Chapter 6 offers a detailed exploration of personality structures that often underpin persistent alienating behaviour. By recognising these patterns, you can adjust your expectations, protect your own mental health, and develop more targeted, protective strategies for your child.

Ultimately, no matter who your co-parent is, your role remains the same: to be the grounded, emotionally safe anchor in your child's world. Understanding the nature of the other parent helps you do that with greater clarity and strength.

ADVICE FOR CHILDREN AND YOUNG PEOPLE EXPERIENCING SEPARATION AND ALIENATION (WRITTEN FOR KIDS)

Separation can be a weird and confusing time for children. It often brings changes to routines, where you live, and relationships, not just with parents but with other family members and even friends. When there is also the pressure of feeling "caught in the middle" or being told not to like one parent, the toll can be huge. This section gives advice aimed at helping children and young people with these challenges to find their voice and stay connected to their own feelings and truths.

You Are Not to Blame

The most important thing to remember is this: none of this is your fault. Parents sometimes stop living together because they can't get along anymore. That is about grown-up problems, *not anything you did*. It is normal to feel sad, angry, or confused, but never feel like you are to blame. You deserve to feel loved and cared for by both parents, even if they don't get along with each other.

It's Okay to Love Both Parents

Sometimes, one parent might make you feel like you have to choose between them and the other. You might hear bad things said about the other parent, or feel worried that someone will get upset if you miss or want to see them. *But it's okay to love* both *of your parents.* You don't have to pick sides. You are allowed to care about and spend time with both, and that doesn't mean you're hurting anyone's feelings.

Feelings Can Be Messy – That's Okay

You might feel lots of different things all at once. Maybe you're happy to see one parent but sad to leave the other. Maybe you're angry one day and missing them the next. *That's all normal.* Feelings can be confusing, especially when things are changing. What matters is giving yourself permission to feel whatever you feel. You don't have to hide it, and you don't have to figure it all out straight away.

You Can Talk to Someone You Trust

Keeping big feelings or worries inside can make you feel worse. If something is bothering you, like feeling stuck between your parents or being told things about the other parent that don't feel right, it's really helpful to talk to someone you trust. This could be:

- A teacher
- A school counsellor
- A family member
- A therapist or support worker
- A helpline for children and young people

Talking doesn't mean you're getting someone in trouble. It means you're *getting help for you,* and that matters.

Sometimes a Parent Is Trying to Keep You Safe

Sometimes, a parent might stop you from seeing the other parent because they're worried about your safety. This can happen if there are serious problems, like violence or harm. If that's the case, they're not trying to be mean or make things harder for you; they're trying to protect you.

But even when someone is trying to keep you safe, it can still feel really confusing or upsetting. You might feel angry, sad, or like you don't understand what's going on. You might even feel stuck in the middle.

If something feels wrong, or if you're not sure what to believe, it's okay to *talk to someone you trust*. They can help you understand what's going on in a way that makes sense and feels fair.

You're not doing anything wrong by asking questions or wanting to know the truth. You're just being brave, and that's a really good thing.

Ask Questions – You Deserve Answers

Sometimes adults tell you things that feel scary or upsetting, especially about the other parent. But you are allowed to ask questions. If something doesn't make sense or feels different from what *you* remember, *it's okay to wonder about it*. You don't have to believe everything just because a grown-up says it. Trust your own memories and feelings, and talk to someone if you're unsure.

Stay Connected in Your Own Way

Even if you're not seeing one parent right now, that doesn't mean they're not still part of your life. You can think about them, remember fun times, look at photos, write letters, or even talk about them with someone you trust. *Staying connected doesn't always mean being in the same room*; it can be about keeping a place for them in your heart until you're ready (or able) to reconnect.

Look After Your Mind and Body

Feeling stuck in the middle of grown-up problems can be stressful. It can make your tummy hurt, mess with your sleep, or make you feel angry or sad a lot of the time. That's why it's so important to take care of yourself. You can:

- Draw, paint, or write down your thoughts
- Go for a walk or do something active
- Listen to music you love
- Talk to a friend who makes you feel better
- Take deep breaths when things feel too big

You don't have to go through this alone. There are people who want to help, and there are things you can do to help yourself feel stronger, bit by bit.

You Have a Voice – And It Matters

Even though you're a child or young person, what you think and feel *really* matters. You have the right to speak up if something doesn't feel okay. If a parent is being mean about the other parent, or trying to make you choose sides, it's okay to say, "I don't like that," or "Please don't talk about them like that." You're allowed to set boundaries, just like grown-ups do.

You don't have to keep secrets that make you uncomfortable. You don't have to take care of your parent's feelings. And you *definitely* don't have to stop loving someone just because someone else says so.

You are allowed to love both your parents. You are allowed to miss someone. You are allowed to want things to feel better. No one can take that away from you.

And remember, if you ever feel stuck or unsure, remember this: your voice matters. And there are people who will listen, believe you, and help.

ADVICE FOR PROFESSIONALS WORKING WITH FAMILIES EXPERIENCING SEPARATION AND EARLY ALIENATION

Professionals who engage with families, whether in education, social care, or mental health, often find themselves at the front line of family change, distress, and conflict. While some cases involve straightforward post-separation adjustments, others may show early signs of PA. Early intervention in these cases can make a critical difference.

This section outlines key principles for professional engagement with children and families during the early stages of alienation risk. It is grounded in trauma-informed, attachment-aware, and system-sensitive practice.

Recognise the Early Signs of Alienation

Children caught in alienation dynamics may present in subtle but distinct ways. Look for:

- Sudden, rigid rejection of one parent without specific, proportionate reasons
- Over-identification with one parent's narrative or language
- Adult-like criticisms of the rejected parent, sometimes mimicking courtroom language
- Apparent lack of ambivalence (i.e., idealisation of one parent, total rejection of the other)
- Involvement in adult matters (e.g., legal issues, allegations, financial grievances)

While these signs are not diagnostic on their own, they should prompt careful, open-minded enquiry, especially when coupled with high parental conflict or previous relational closeness to the rejected parent.

Maintain a Child-Centred and Neutral Stance

Children experiencing alienation are often placed in loyalty binds, feeling pressure to side with one parent at the cost of the other. Professionals must:

- Avoid reinforcing polarised narratives (e.g., "good" vs "bad" parent)
- Be cautious about assuming that the most emotionally expressive parent is the most truthful
- Reassure the child that they are allowed to love and miss both parents
- Support the child's voice, while being sensitive to how that voice may have been influenced

Neutrality does not mean passivity; it means being an advocate for the child's *right to relational safety and integrity.*

Understand Alienation as a Relational, Not Individual, Problem

Avoid pathologising the child or blaming one parent without a full contextual understanding. Alienation is typically the product not of individual pathology but of relational patterns, systemic conflict, and often unaddressed trauma.

- Use frameworks that account for family systems, attachment disruption, and emotional manipulation
- Consider how the child's narrative may be shaped by fear, guilt, or emotional dependency, not just conscious choice
- Explore the relational histories and broader ecology around the child before drawing conclusions.

Support Relational Repair Where Appropriate

Early intervention can help prevent the solidification of alienation. Professionals can:

- Encourage and support safe, meaningful contact with both parents where there is no evidence of abuse
- Help children express ambivalent feelings without pressure to choose sides
- Work with both parents (separately or jointly) to improve communication, emotional regulation, and child-focused thinking

For teachers, this may involve validating the child's feelings and working with both caregivers. For mental health professionals, it may involve early, gentle forms of reunification work. For social workers, it may mean initiating dialogue around contact and co-parenting before formal safeguarding thresholds are crossed.

Avoid Becoming Part of the Triangulation

Professionals are sometimes unwittingly drawn into the dynamics of alienation. One parent may try to:

- Enlist professionals to "validate" their view of the other parent
- Selectively share information to position themselves as the safer or more appropriate caregiver
- Criticise other professionals who have not taken their side

Remain mindful of these dynamics and keep the focus on the child's experience and needs. This includes:

- Seeking corroboration from multiple sources
- Being wary of adopting language that mirrors parental narratives
- Avoiding actions or documentation that inadvertently endorse rejection without balanced assessment

Use Your Role to Create Protective Space

Whether you are a teacher, therapist, or support worker, your relationship with the child can become a protective buffer. You can:

- Provide a stable space where the child feels seen and safe
- Reinforce the child's autonomy and permission to care for both parents
- Challenge binary or extreme narratives gently and supportively
- Offer a model of emotional regulation and empathy

Collaborate with Other Professionals

Alienation often sits below formal thresholds of child protection but above typical post-separation adjustment. Collaboration across services can help:

- Monitor emerging patterns without overreacting to a single report
- Share information appropriately (with consent) to build a holistic picture
- Avoid fragmentation and contradictory messaging to the family

Early-stage multi-agency work can prevent entrenchment and help families access resources that promote relational repair rather than adversarial escalation.

ENGAGING IN CRITICAL ENQUIRY

Professionals working with families affected by separation and potential alienation must approach each case with *critical enquiry*, not passive acceptance. Too often, practitioners unwittingly reinforce alienating dynamics by uncritically adopting the narrative of the aligned parent, particularly when it is delivered with emotional intensity or apparent coherence. This is especially dangerous when the child's stated views and preferences closely echo that parent's script. While the voice of the child is a vital part of any assessment, it must be understood *in context* and never accepted at face value without robust exploration.

Alienation is a form of psychological abuse. It distorts the child's perceptions, feelings, and memories, often without the child being aware that this is happening. When a child presents with unjustified rejection of one parent, professionals must ask, "Why is this child saying this?" "Who benefits from this narrative?" and "What relational dynamics lie beneath the surface?" Failure to do so may lead to outcomes that deepen the child's trauma and compound the fracture of the family system. Engaging in critical enquiry means:

- Seeking evidence beyond surface narratives
- Exploring all relational histories and power dynamics
- Considering the possibility of psychological manipulation, just as one would consider physical or emotional abuse
- Understanding that a child's *voice* may, in some cases, be a *ventriloquised script*, shaped by fear, guilt, or enmeshment

Just as no professional would ignore signs of domestic violence or coercive control, the same level of vigilance must be applied when alienation is suspected. To uncritically endorse the views of one parent, or of a child whose expressions have been shaped by alienating behaviours, is not neutrality. It is complicity in harm.

Children do not need professionals to validate distorted realities. They need professionals who are willing to *pause, investigate, and think systemically*. They need adults who can hold complexity, challenge bias, and make decisions grounded not just in what is said but in what is *true*.

In short: support the whole family system. Investigate thoroughly. And make decisions based not on appearance but on evidence, and on what genuinely serves the child's long-term relational and psychological wellbeing.

SUMMARY

This chapter has offered practical, trauma-informed guidance for parents, children, and professionals navigating the early stages of separation and potential alienation. It emphasised the importance of preserving secure relationships, validating children's emotions without reinforcing polarised narratives, and intervening early when signs of unjustified rejection appear. For professionals, it underscored the need for critical enquiry and systemic thinking, challenging the automatic acceptance of dominant narratives, including the child's voice when it may have been shaped by manipulation. Protecting children in these contexts requires thoughtful, evidence-based responses that prioritise relational safety, challenge distorted dynamics, and support the child's long-term psychological wellbeing.

BIBLIOGRAPHY

Brazelton, T. B., & Greenspan, S. I. (2000). *The irreducible needs of children: What every child must have to grow, learn, and flourish.* Perseus Publishing.

Brown, C. (2024). *Effective co-parenting or parallel parenting with a narcissist: Set boundaries, eliminate conflict, protect yourself, and raise emotionally secure children.* Independently Published.

Carter, W. (2023). *Parallel parenting.* Independently Published.

Dean, A. (2024). *Choosing yourself when your parents separate.* The Centre for Childhood Relational Trauma.

Hine, B. A. (2023). *Parental alienation: A contemporary guide for parents, practitioners, and policymakers.* Independently Published.

Fosters, T. R. (2024). *Emotional regulation for parents: Actionable strategies and mindfulness techniques to understand triggers, reduce household conflict, and build stronger family bonds.* Independently Published.

Johnson, E. (2024). *The 50/50 solution: The surprisingly simple choice that makes moms, dads, and kids happier and healthier after a split.* Sourcebooks.

Leving, J. M. (2007). *Divorce wars: A field guide to winning tactics, preemptive strikes, and top maneuvers when divorce gets ugly.* HarperCollins.

Leving, J. M. (2012). *How to be a good divorced dad.* Jossey—Bass.

McGhee, C. (2011). *Parenting apart: How separated and divorced parents can raise happy and secure kids.* Vermilion.

Parenting After Parting Committee. (2024). *Parenting through separation: Putting children first* (2nd ed.). Resolution.

Shaoul, M. (2025). *The co-parenting method: Six steps to raise happy kids after separation and divorce.* Vermilion.

Wolfe, H. (2025). *Practical co-parenting with a narcissist: Empowering strategies to survive toxic abuse, reduce conflict and set boundaries to protect yourself and raise emotionally healthy children.* Independently Published.

Wolfkill, M. (2024). *Co-parenting with a narcissist: A life-changing guide to protect your child, set strong boundaries, and keep your sanity after divorcing a narcissistic ex.* Independently Published.

Woodall, K., & Woodall, N. (2007). *The guide for separated parents: Putting children first.* Piatkus Books.

15

PARENTAL ALIENATION IN THE COURTS

While it is always hoped that separating parents can prioritise their child's wellbeing and resolve disputes amicably, the reality is that, in many high-conflict separations, this becomes untenable. In such cases, legal intervention is not only necessary but also unavoidable. Family courts thus become a central arena where PA is not just revealed but also often intensified. The adversarial nature of legal proceedings can also entrench polarised narratives, reinforce power imbalances, and amplify the strategies used by alienating parents, sometimes even legitimising them under the guise of protective concern or custodial preference.

As such, PA increasingly surfaces as a key issue in courtrooms across many jurisdictions, particularly in cases involving contact disputes and custody arrangements. Yet, despite growing scholarly consensus on PA as a form of psychological abuse and post-separation coercive control, courts have not always responded consistently or effectively. Legal systems can struggle to distinguish PA from justified estrangement, particularly in the absence of clear guidelines, rigorous assessments, or adequately trained professionals. As such, PA cases are not only legally complex; they are ethically fraught, psychologically nuanced, and procedurally challenging.

This chapter offers an in-depth exploration of how PA is understood, addressed, and, at times, mishandled within family court settings. It examines prevailing legal frameworks and practices, highlighting the structural and cultural factors that shape judicial responses to alienation. Attention is

DOI: 10.4324/9781003630944-20

given to the role of expert witnesses, psychological evaluations, and evidentiary standards, as well as the critical importance, and difficulty, of incorporating children's voices meaningfully and safely.

Author's Note: This chapter is intended to provide contextual insight into the legal handling of parental alienation but is not a substitute for legal advice. Legal frameworks vary by jurisdiction, and readers are encouraged to seek qualified legal counsel within their own countries.

LEGAL RIGHTS AND RESPONSIBILITIES OF PARENTS POST-SEPARATION: A GLOBAL OVERVIEW

In the aftermath of separation or divorce, the legal recognition of parental rights and responsibilities varies widely across jurisdictions. Yet, a common thread unites many legal systems: the commitment to uphold the best interests of the child as the guiding principle in post-separation arrangements. While the specifics differ from country to country, most legal frameworks seek to balance parental autonomy with the child's right to maintain meaningful relationships with both parents, an aim that can become significantly complicated in the presence of PA.

Globally, there is a general recognition that both parents retain certain duties and entitlements following separation. These typically include financial obligations (such as child support), legal authority over major decisions affecting the child (e.g., education, health, and religion), and the right to maintain regular contact with the child. However, the extent to which these rights are protected, enforced, or susceptible to manipulation varies significantly.

In countries such as *Canada*, *Australia*, and several *European Union* member states, there is a strong legal emphasis on shared parental responsibility, even when physical custody is not equally distributed. These jurisdictions often adopt a presumption that both parents should remain involved in the child's life unless there is evidence to suggest that such involvement would pose a risk to the child's well-being. In such systems, the courts may grant joint legal custody (decision-making authority) even when the child primarily resides with one parent.

In contrast, countries like *Japan*, *India*, and, historically, *South Korea* operate under legal frameworks that typically award sole custody to one parent, often the mother, with limited or non-enforceable contact rights for the non-custodial parent. This has contributed to widespread concerns about the institutionalisation of parent–child bond disruption, especially in cases where the custodial parent actively restricts access.

Brazil represents a unique example, having explicitly legislated against PA through federal law, recognising it as a form of psychological abuse. The law mandates psychological evaluation and allows for judicial intervention in cases of confirmed alienation. However, the application of this law has sparked debate, particularly concerning its use in high-conflict or abusive contexts.

In *the United States*, family law is state-specific, leading to wide variation in how parental responsibilities are allocated. Nevertheless, many states now acknowledge PA as a factor in custody decisions, and some provide statutory remedies, including court-ordered therapy or changes in custody. Likewise, *South Africa's* Children's Act, while not naming PA explicitly, frames the child's best interests as paramount and has increasingly accommodated interventions in alienation cases.

Importantly, legal concepts such as *parental responsibility, custodial rights,* and *contact orders* may carry different meanings depending on the jurisdictional context. In some systems, parental responsibility encompasses not only legal authority but also a moral duty to sustain the parent–child bond. This may include an implicit obligation not to undermine the child's relationship with the other parent, a duty that is easily eroded when PA occurs undetected or unaddressed.

Yet, even in progressive systems, the enforcement of contact and custody orders remains inconsistent. Legal remedies can be slow, resource-intensive, or ineffectual, particularly when the alienating parent is skilled at manipulating narratives around child welfare or protection. Moreover, courts may lack training or clarity on how to differentiate between justified estrangement and alienation, an ambiguity that is exploited in high-conflict cases.

However, across jurisdictions, it is increasingly recognised that maintaining post-separation parental involvement is critical to child development. This principle must be actively safeguarded through legal and procedural clarity, interdisciplinary expertise, and cultural sensitivity. As global understanding of PA deepens, legal systems must evolve not only to respond to its manifestations but also to anticipate and prevent its occurrence by embedding the protection of parent–child relationships more robustly into post-separation family law.

WHAT COURTS SHOULD DO IN CASES OF PARENTAL ALIENATION

The legal system holds both the authority and the ethical obligation to act in the best interests of children, particularly in situations where one parent is engaging in behaviours that intentionally disrupt or sever the child's bond with the other. Although legal frameworks differ considerably across jurisdictions, there are key principles that should guide the family court's approach to PA, especially as the phenomenon becomes more widely recognised as a form of psychological abuse and post-separation coercive control.

Acknowledge PA as a Valid and Distinct Form of Harm

The first step is recognising PA not simply as a contact dispute or a manifestation of high-conflict parenting but also as a distinct form of relational harm that can have severe psychological consequences for the child and the targeted parent. In jurisdictions where PA is not yet formally codified in law, courts can still draw upon existing provisions related to emotional abuse, child welfare, and psychological harm to identify alienating behaviours and respond appropriately.

Judges, legal professionals, and child welfare assessors must also be equipped to distinguish PA from justified estrangement or legitimate protective concerns. This requires specific training and a multi-disciplinary understanding of the patterns and consequences of alienating behaviours.

Conduct Robust, Evidence-Informed Assessments

In cases where PA is alleged, courts should not rely on surface-level narratives or one-sided allegations. Instead, they must ensure that comprehensive, evidence-based assessments are conducted by suitably qualified professionals. These evaluations should apply empirically validated models, such as the Five-Factor Model for PA assessment, and involve input from all relevant parties, including the child, both parents, and any collateral sources.

It is essential that evaluators are free from bias, receive specialised training in PA and family systems trauma, and are held to high standards of forensic integrity.

Prioritise the Child's Long-Term Psychological Health

While the child's expressed wishes should be considered, courts must differentiate between authentic preferences and those shaped by manipulation or fear. In cases of PA, the child's rejection of a once-loved parent is often a symptom of coercive dynamics rather than an autonomous decision. The legal system has a duty to look beneath the surface and protect the child's long-term well-being, even when this means taking actions contrary to their current stated preferences.

Implement Targeted, Proportionate Interventions

Where PA is confirmed or strongly indicated, courts should consider a graduated set of interventions based on the severity and persistence of the alienation (see Chapter 17). These may include:

- *Reunification programmes* involving specialised therapy for the child and both parents
- *Sanctions* for non-compliance with court orders, including financial penalties or, in extreme cases, custody reversal
- *Supervised contact* to rebuild the parent–child relationship in a safe and structured environment

- *Parental education* and behavioural change programmes for the alienating parent

Interventions must be trauma-informed, child-focused, and subject to ongoing review to ensure that they are having the intended effect and not inadvertently exacerbating the alienation.

Ensure Enforcement Mechanisms Are Credible and Swift

A frequent failure in PA cases is the inadequate enforcement of existing court orders. Delays, non-compliance, and procedural ambiguities enable alienating behaviours to continue unchecked. Courts must establish clear timelines, monitoring processes, and consequences for breach, sending a strong message that undermining a child's relationship with a parent will not be tolerated.

Support Legal Advocacy for Targeted Parents

Legal professionals representing targeted parents play a critical role in educating the court, presenting evidence effectively, and ensuring the parents' rights are not further eroded by procedural delays or biased assumptions. In systems where PA is not yet recognised, these advocates often carry the burden of making the issue visible within a sceptical or uninformed legal environment.

To function ethically and effectively, courts should ensure that all parties, especially children and targeted parents, have access to fair representation and informed advocacy.

CURRENT UNDERSTANDING ON PARENTAL ALIENATION IN COURT

PA has become an increasingly prominent, and polarising, topic within family court litigation globally. While its recognition has grown within legal and clinical circles, its interpretation, admissibility, and application remain subjects of significant debate. The complexity of the issue is compounded by its intersections with domestic violence (DV), gender dynamics, and inconsistent forensic practices, resulting in wide variation in how PA is understood and operationalised in courts across jurisdictions.

Diverging Interpretations: Misuse or Misunderstanding?

A dominant critique, particularly prominent in North American discourse, is that PA is frequently invoked not as a genuine concern but as a tactical counterclaim, most often by fathers, against mothers' allegations of abuse. Scholars such as Meier and Milchman argue that the court system has, in some cases, become complicit in "invisibilising" male violence by accepting alienation claims without rigorous scrutiny. This concern has been echoed in qualitative research in which survivor-mothers reported feeling re-victimised by the legal system and were often reluctant to disclose abuse due to fear of alienation counterclaims.

These critiques gained further traction following a 2023 report to the United Nations Special Rapporteur on violence against women, which argued that the concept of PA was routinely weaponised against women, particularly in custody disputes involving allegations of sexual abuse. Concerns have also been raised about the reliability and qualifications of self-declared PA experts, and the lack of regulation in how expert testimony is deployed in court.

However, this perspective is far from universally accepted. Other large-scale case reviews, such as those by Lorandos and colleagues, challenge the notion that PA claims function primarily as tools of abuse. These reviews found no cases in which custody was awarded to a demonstrably abusive parent following a PA claim. Moreover, they found that parents, regardless of gender, who were found to have engaged in alienating behaviours were more likely to lose parenting time. Importantly, they also observed that PA claims and DV claims were not mutually exclusive. In many cases, both forms of abuse were found to co-exist, with PA emerging as part of a broader pattern of coercive and controlling behaviour.

Such findings underscore the need to move beyond binary, gendered narratives and towards a more empirically grounded understanding of family dynamics. It is unequivocally the case that both false PA claims and false DV claims are made by both mothers and fathers. Mischaracterising either phenomenon as gender-specific not only undermines the credibility of the legal process but also compromises child safety and the integrity of judicial decision-making.

Global Echoes: The Case of Brazil, Spain, Canada, and the UK

These tensions are not confined to the United States. In *Brazil*, where PA is legally recognised and penalised under federal law, critics argue that the concept has, at times, been misused to delegitimise valid abuse claims, particularly in high-conflict custody disputes. The absence of clear, evidence-based evaluative procedures has left courts vulnerable to subjective interpretation, a concern echoed in *Spain*, where judicial decisions on PA often hinge more on courtroom advocacy and judicial leanings than on robust clinical assessments.

In *Canada*, the situation is similarly ambiguous. While there is growing recognition of PA, qualitative research shows that some women in domestic violence shelters are fearful of raising abuse claims in court, anticipating that these will be met with alienation counterclaims. Yet case reviews offer mixed conclusions: some suggest that DV claims are taken seriously, while others find the opposite. Both sides converge on a common point: the need for deeper understanding and training among legal professionals regarding the nuanced relationship between alienation and family violence.

The *UK* presents an additional layer of complexity due to the inaccessibility of court records and limited empirical research. Small-scale qualitative studies suggest that some mothers fear raising abuse claims for fear of retaliation via PA accusations. Conversely, other research indicates that many fathers experience systemic bias within the family court, including the dismissal of their own claims of alienation and abuse, and a general devaluation of their parental role.

These contradictory findings reflect an unresolved tension: how to uphold the legal commitment to child welfare and meaningful parental relationships without enabling the misuse of PA as a litigation strategy, or, conversely, the erasure of real alienation dynamics under the presumption that they are always defensive or manipulative in nature.

The Real Issue: Conceptual and Procedural Uncertainty

What emerges across jurisdictions is not a lack of concern about PA, but rather a lack of conceptual clarity and procedural consistency. There remains insufficient empirical insight into:

- *How and when* claims of PA and DV are brought forward;
- *How legitimacy* is determined, and whether current assessments are valid;
- *What outcomes* these determinations lead to, and whether they align with the best interests of the child.

Too often, decisions are made based on incomplete or biased evaluations, poorly defined terms, or adversarial court practices that entrench, rather than resolve, familial conflict. In jurisdictions where PA is recognised, its interpretation can still vary drastically depending on judicial discretion, evidentiary standards, and the availability, or lack, of qualified expert testimony.

Moreover, courts across the globe are still navigating the tension between the "pro-contact" principle (the presumption that children benefit from contact with both parents) and the need to protect children from genuine harm, including both PA and other forms of abuse. This balancing act is often performed without the necessary tools to distinguish coercion from legitimate concern, or trauma-induced estrangement from strategic alienation.

INCORPORATING CHILDREN'S VIEWS AND ASSOCIATED CHALLENGES IN FAMILY COURT PROCEEDINGS

The inclusion of the child's voice in family court proceedings is a widely endorsed principle, grounded in both ethical commitments to child-centred practice and international legal obligations such as the United Nations Convention on the Rights of the Child (UNCRC). Children have the right to express their views in matters affecting them, and those views should be given due weight in accordance with their age and maturity. However, in cases involving PA, the implementation of this principle becomes acutely challenging.

The Paradox of the Child's Voice in Alienation Cases

In PA cases, a core tension emerges: while the child's perspective is vital, it may be significantly shaped, or even wholly manufactured, by the alienating parent. The child may articulate a strong and unequivocal rejection of one parent, which the court is then called upon to interpret. However, unlike in other child custody disputes, the child's views in PA scenarios cannot be taken at face value without a deeper interrogation of their context and origin.

This presents a fundamental paradox: courts must respect the child's voice without assuming its authenticity. This requires not just careful listening but informed, psychologically attuned interpretation. The challenge is not simply one of eliciting the child's views but of discerning their meaning.

The Mechanisms and Risks of Influence

Children exposed to alienating behaviours may internalise distorted narratives about the targeted parent. Over time, they may come to believe these narratives as their own, making them highly convincing to professionals who lack specific training in PA dynamics. The alienating parent's influence may not be overtly coercive; it may be subtle, persistent, and embedded in day-to-day interactions and emotional cues that are invisible to outsiders. This can result in what appears to be a competent, autonomous expression of will when, in fact, it is the product of psychological manipulation.

Compounding the issue, children may also feel an intense loyalty to the alienating parent, fearing rejection or emotional withdrawal if they express affection or a desire for contact with the targeted parent. In this context, what is presented as the child's "voice" may actually be a survival strategy, shaped by the implicit threat of emotional abandonment.

Professional Interpretation and the Role of Training

The critical task for courts and professionals, therefore, is not to disregard the child's voice but to contextualise it. This requires a high level of professional expertise and a trauma-informed understanding of how PA operates. Social workers, psychologists, and child welfare assessors must be equipped to distinguish between genuine expressions of distress and those that are symptomatic of coercion or enmeshment.

Training in PA dynamics is essential. Without it, professionals may mistake trauma-bonded allegiance to the alienating parent for authentic preference, or misinterpret the targeted parent's distress and frustration as signs of instability or hostility. The consequences of such misinterpretations can be profound, resulting in judicial decisions that entrench, rather than mitigate, the harm of alienation.

Evaluative Techniques and Methodological Cautions

Assessing a child's views in the context of PA should involve multiple sources of information and longitudinal observation wherever possible. Techniques may include structured interviews, behavioural observation, collateral input from schools or extended family, and attachment-based assessments. Indirect methods, such as play-based evaluations or narrative techniques, can be valuable in younger children; however, these must be interpreted with great care and clinical insight.

Ultimately, courts must recognise that expressed preferences are not always synonymous with best interests. While children's perspectives must be heard, they must also be held within a wider evidentiary and psychological framework that accounts for the distorting effects of alienation.

Striking a Developmentally Appropriate Balance

The goal is not to silence the child but to protect the child from being placed in a position of undue influence or moral responsibility. Children, especially older children, may present with what appear to be firm convictions about rejecting a parent. However, the apparent maturity of these convictions does not necessarily correlate with emotional independence or informed decision-making. Where PA is suspected or substantiated, courts must remain vigilant to the possibility that the child's voice, however clear, may be carrying someone else's message.

ADDITIONAL CHALLENGES IN PARENTAL ALIENATION CASES

Several other persistent challenges hinder accurate identification and fair adjudication in court. These difficulties stem from systemic gaps in knowledge, cultural assumptions, and the adversarial nature of family law proceedings.

Limited Professional Understanding and Scepticism

One of the most pressing issues is that many legal and mental health professionals still possess a limited understanding of PA or remain sceptical of its validity. This lack of awareness can severely disadvantage targeted parents, particularly when allegations of alienation are misunderstood as simple high-conflict parenting or as tactical deflection from more serious allegations. In such environments, parents raising legitimate concerns about PA may find themselves dismissed or discredited.

Gender Bias in Judicial Interpretation

Gender bias continues to permeate family court processes. Stereotypical views of mothers as default primary caregivers and fathers as secondary or less nurturing can shape assumptions about who is more likely to be the alienating or abusive parent. Fathers who report being targeted by PA often encounter significant scepticism, in part because societal narratives frequently minimise male victimhood. Conversely, mothers may struggle to be believed when PA is claimed against them, especially in the context of prior allegations of abuse. These biases can distort the interpretation of behaviour and influence judicial outcomes in ways that are not aligned with the child's best interests.

Expectation Bias and Misinterpretation of Vulnerability

Professional decision-making is also affected by expectation bias, namely assumptions about how a "normal" or "credible" parent or child ought to behave. Parents who are neurodivergent, experiencing mental health challenges, or survivors of trauma may present in ways that deviate from these expectations, leading to misinterpretation of their behaviour as erratic, harmful, or unfit. Such assessments may be based more on perceived deviance from normative parenting scripts than on any substantiated risk to the child.

Courtroom Manipulation by the Alienating Parent

Alienating parents often present convincingly in court, adept at shaping narratives that portray them as victims while casting the targeted parent as unstable, abusive, or disengaged. This capacity for manipulation, especially in systems lacking forensic scrutiny or standardised evaluation, can result in misplaced judicial sympathy and flawed custody decisions. False allegations of abuse, when unchecked, can both derail proceedings and inflict severe reputational harm on the targeted parent.

Complexity of High-Conflict Cases

PA frequently emerges in the context of entrenched, high-conflict custody disputes, where the emotional volatility and strategic hostility between parents make it exceedingly difficult to disentangle truth from perception. In these cases, the court must navigate competing narratives, unclear timelines, and a child who may appear legitimately distressed, yet whose distress may stem from psychological coercion rather than lived harm. Without comprehensive, multi-perspective assessments, the risk of misjudging such dynamics remains high.

EXPERT WITNESSES AND EVALUATIONS

Expert witnesses and court-appointed evaluations play a pivotal role in the legal response to PA. As courts grapple with the complex psychological dynamics at play, especially in high-conflict custody disputes, expert input is often relied upon to provide clarity, credibility, and context. However, while these inputs can be invaluable, they also raise serious concerns regarding consistency, quality, regulation, and potential bias.

The Role of Expert Witnesses

In PA cases, expert witnesses, typically psychologists, psychiatrists, or therapists, are tasked with translating psychological complexity into judicially actionable insight. Their remit may include identifying signs of alienation, distinguishing it from justified estrangement or loyalty conflict, assessing attachment patterns, and recommending interventions such as reunification therapy or therapeutic supervision. Their testimony can significantly influence custody outcomes and contact arrangements, making their role both powerful and ethically fraught.

These professionals must also serve as neutral educators to the court, explaining how alienating behaviours manifest, how they affect child development, and how family systems can become enmeshed in dynamics that the court may not immediately recognise. When done well, such testimony provides the court with the nuanced understanding necessary to act in the child's long-term best interests.

Psychological and Custody Evaluations

Courts may commission comprehensive evaluations to examine the family's psychosocial environment. These assessments typically involve multiple interviews (with parents, children, and sometimes extended family or other collateral sources), behavioural observations, standardised measures, and review of documents such as therapy notes, school records, or prior legal filings. Properly conducted, these evaluations can help courts identify patterns of coercive control, manipulation, or emotional harm that may not be evident from legal pleadings alone.

However, evaluations are only as robust as the professionals who conduct them. Without clear standards for how PA assessments should be undertaken, and without mandatory training in PA-specific dynamics, these evaluations may reflect the biases or theoretical leanings of the evaluator more than the facts of the case.

Challenges and Controversies

The use of expert witnesses and evaluations in PA cases is not without serious concerns. First, there is no universally accepted regulatory framework for qualifying someone as a PA expert. Many jurisdictions do not require specific certification or training in PA for an individual to present as an expert witness. This leads to wide variability in quality, methodology, and credibility. In some cases, self-declared experts have provided testimony that lacks empirical support or is grounded in outdated or discredited theories.

Second, the adversarial nature of family court proceedings can compromise the integrity of expert input. Experts may be perceived, rightly or wrongly, as aligned with the party that commissioned them. This undermines their perceived neutrality and can exacerbate tensions, especially in cases already characterised by high levels of mistrust.

Third, personal bias and theoretical orientation can shape the interpretation of data. An evaluator who dismisses PA as a valid construct may fail to detect genuine alienation. Conversely, an evaluator overly focused on identifying PA may misinterpret justified estrangement as manipulation. In both cases, the child's welfare is placed at risk.

Fourth, the emotional toll and logistical burden of evaluations cannot be overlooked. These processes are often long, intrusive, and expensive, and they may deepen existing conflict. For children, repeated interviews and psychological assessments can be confusing or distressing, particularly if their views are misrepresented or misunderstood.

The Need for Reform

Given these concerns, there is a growing consensus that courts require better safeguards and clearer standards around the use of expert evidence in PA cases. These include:

- Establishing minimum qualifications and PA-specific training for expert witnesses;
- Developing standardised protocols for PA assessments based on validated models;
- Encouraging the use of court-appointed, neutral evaluators rather than partisan experts;
- Providing judicial training to help judges critically assess expert testimony;
- Promoting peer review and accountability mechanisms for evaluators who work in high-stakes custody disputes.

Without such reforms, courts risk making life-altering decisions based on inconsistent or flawed testimony, thereby failing to meet the standard of acting in the child's best interests.

SUMMARY

This chapter critically examined how PA is approached within family court proceedings across global jurisdictions. It explored how legal rights and responsibilities are structured post-separation and how the concept of PA is variably recognised and adjudicated across different legal systems. The chapter outlined what courts *should* do when faced with PA, recognising its distinct psychological harms, implementing evidence-based assessments, and prioritising the long-term well-being of the child, even where expressed preferences may be shaped by coercive dynamics. However, what is currently happening in many courts often falls short of these ideals. Competing academic interpretations, gendered assumptions, and variable legal responses have contributed to inconsistent outcomes and, in some cases, harm to children and targeted parents.

A central challenge lies in balancing the imperative to include the child's voice with the need to evaluate its authenticity in the context of potential manipulation. The chapter further addressed additional systemic challenges, including professional scepticism about PA, gender and expectation bias, and the often problematic use of expert witnesses and evaluations in contested custody cases. It underscored that while expert input is essential, the lack of regulation, inconsistent methodologies, and susceptibility to adversarial pressures can compromise both the fairness and efficacy of court decisions.

Looking ahead, a series of critical reforms can be identified to enhance the legal system's handling of PA. These include early intervention, improved training for legal professionals, and the development of more robust, interdisciplinary, and trauma-informed assessment processes. Calls are already being made for specialised judges, consistent enforcement of court orders, better integration between family and criminal courts, and a renewed emphasis on the child's best interests, not merely in principle but in practice. While reforms must be tailored to the jurisdictional context, the shared objective must be a more responsive, equitable, and empirically grounded approach to parental alienation within the family justice system.

BIBLIOGRAPHY

Alsalem, R. (2023). *Custody, violence against women and violence against children*. https://documents-dds-ny.un.org/doc/UNDOC/GEN/G23/070/18/PDF/G2307018.pdf?OpenElement

Barnett, A. (2020). A genealogy of hostility: Parental alienation in England and Wales. *Journal of Social Welfare & Family Law*, *42*, 18–29. https://doi.org/10.1080/09649069.2019.1701921

Birchall, J., & Choudhry, S. (2022). 'I was punished for telling the truth': How allegations of parental alienation are used to silence, sideline and disempower survivors of domestic abuse in family law proceedings. *Journal of Gender-Based Violence*. https://doi.org/10.1332/239868021X16287966471815

Birnbaum, R., & Bala, N. (2024). A retrospective study of outcomes of custody reversal in parental alienation cases. *UNBLJ*, *75*, 62.

Casas Vila, G. (2020). Parental alienation syndrome in Spain: Opposed by the government but accepted in the courts. *Journal of Social Welfare and Family Law*, *42*(1), 45–55. https://doi.org/10.1080/09649069.2019.1701923

Clemente, M., & Padilla-Racero, D. (2021). Obey the justice system or protect children? The moral dilemma posed by false parental alienation syndrome. *Children and Youth Services Review*, *120*, 105728. https://doi.org/10.1016/j.childyouth.2020.105728

Gutowski, E., & Goodman, L. A. (2020). "Like I'm Invisible": IPV survivor-mothers' perceptions of seeking child custody through the family court system. *Journal of Family Violence, 35*, 441–457. https://doi.org/10.1007/s10896-019-00063-1

Harman, J. J., & Lorandos, D. (2021). Allegations of family violence in court: How parental alienation affects judicial outcomes. *Psychology, Public Policy, and Law, 27*(2), 184–208. https://doi.org/10.1037/law0000301

Hine, B. A., Roy, E. M., Huang, C. Y., & Bates, E. (2025). Father's experiences of negotiating co-parenting arrangements and family court. *Social Sciences, 14*(1), 29. https://doi.org/10.3390/socsci14010029

Meier, J. S., Dickson, S., O'Sullivan, C. S., & Rosen, L. N. (2022a). Harman and Lorandos' false critique of Meier et al.'s family court study. *Journal of Family Trauma, Child Custody & Child Development, 19*, 119–138. https://doi.org/10.1080/26904586.2022.2086659

Meier, J. S., Dickson, S., O'Sullivan, C. S., & Rosen, L. N. (2022b). The trouble with Harman and Lorandos' parental alienation in family court study (2020). *Journal of Family Trauma, Child Custody & Child Development*. https://doi.org/10.1080/26904586.2022.2036286

Meier, J. S., Dickson, S., O'Sullivan, C. S., Rosen, L. N., & Hayes, J. (2019). *Child custody outcomes in cases involving parental alienation and abuse allegations* (GWU Law School Public Law Research Paper No. 2019-56). http://dx.doi.org/10.2139/ssrn.3448062

Milchman, M. S. (2024). Oversimplified beliefs about child abuse allegations in custody cases with alienation rebuttals–review of empirical data. *Journal of Family Trauma, Child Custody & Child Development, 21*(2), 165–192. https://doi.org/10.1080/26904586.2024.2307612

Myers, J. E., & Mercer, J. (2022). Parental alienation in family court: Attacking expert testimony. *Barry L Child and Family Law Journal, 10*, 68.

Paquin-Boudreau, A., Poitras, K., & Bala, N. (2022). Family court responses to claims of parental alienation in Quebec. *International Journal of Law, Policy and the Family, 36*. https://doi.org/10.1093/lawfam/ebac014

Rao, A. G. (2021). Rejecting 'unjustified' rejection: Why family courts should exclude parental alienation experts. *Boston College Law Review, 62*, 1759.

Sharples, A., Harman, J. J., & Lorandos, D. (2025). Findings of abuse in families affected by parental alienation. *Journal of Family Violence, 40*, 225–235. https://doi.org/https://doi.org/10.1007/s10896-023-00575-x

Varavei, H., & Harman, J. J. (2025). The illusory correlation between parental alienation and other forms of family violence. *International Journal of Social Welfare, 34*(1), e12692. https://doi.org/10.1111/ijsw.12692

16

ADVICE ON LEGAL PROCESSES

Engaging with the family court system is often one of the most stressful and destabilising experiences for families, particularly in cases involving PA. For targeted parents, the legal process can feel overwhelming and adversarial, compounding the psychological toll of already strained relationships. Children, too, may experience heightened anxiety and confusion, as their voices are drawn into proceedings they may not fully understand. Legal professionals, meanwhile, face the challenge of disentangling complex family dynamics under immense time pressures and within systems that may not be adequately equipped to address PA.

This chapter seeks to provide clear, practical guidance for those directly and indirectly affected by PA. It is divided into three parts. The first section offers advice to parents navigating the challenges of alienation, including strategies for supporting their child while protecting their own wellbeing. The second section turns to children, acknowledging their unique perspective and providing guidance on resilience, coping, and safe avenues for expression. The final section addresses legal professionals, highlighting the importance of awareness, training, and trauma-informed practice in ensuring that cases are approached with fairness, sensitivity, and an unwavering focus on the child's best interests.

By offering targeted advice to these different groups, the chapter aims to reduce the sense of isolation that often accompanies PA and provide

DOI: 10.4324/9781003630944-21

constructive pathways forward in the midst of what is, for many, one of the most difficult journeys of their lives.

THE IMPACT OF FAMILY COURT PROCEEDINGS

Before offering advice to families and professionals, it is essential to acknowledge the profound strain that family court processes impose on those navigating PA. Both parents and children are deeply affected by the adversarial nature of legal proceedings, which can amplify emotional distress, disrupt relationships, and prolong conflict.

Parents' Experiences

For parents, litigation involving PA is often overwhelming, emotionally exhausting, and financially draining. They may be forced to revisit painful histories of conflict and face allegations that challenge their competence and character as caregivers. Parents frequently describe feelings of injustice or bias in the courtroom, particularly if they believe their concerns about PA or abuse have been dismissed. These perceptions can erode trust in the system, reduce willingness to comply with court orders, and deepen hostility between parents.

The quality of legal representation also significantly shapes parents' experiences. Skilled advocacy can help parents navigate the complexities of court, yet not all have access to high-quality legal support. Long delays and multiple hearings further intensify stress and can entrench alienation, as the child's relationship with the targeted parent deteriorates over time. The adversarial nature of proceedings also risks entrenching conflict, making cooperative co-parenting even harder to achieve after the case is concluded.

Children's Experiences

For children, family court involvement can be bewildering and destabilising. The process often exposes them to parental hostility, contradictory narratives, and repeated questioning by unfamiliar professionals. Many children experience anxiety, guilt, or confusion, particularly when pressured to choose sides. Extended litigation can disrupt daily routines, friendships, and schooling, undermining their sense of stability and normalcy.

In PA cases, the impact on children's relationships is especially acute. The bond with the targeted parent may be damaged or severed, depriving them of a source of love and support. At the same time, ongoing exposure to conflict can erode their self-esteem, distort their sense of identity, and leave them vulnerable to long-term psychological consequences, including depression, anxiety, and relational difficulties in adulthood.

Recognising these profound impacts is crucial. Any advice for navigating PA must take into account the heavy toll of legal proceedings, acknowledging that parents and children enter the process already strained and in need of sensitive, informed, and practical support.

ADVICE FOR PARENTS

Navigating the legal system when dealing with PA can be a complex and daunting process. This section aims to provide parents with guidance on how to navigate the family court system, obtain legal representation, and prepare for court proceedings. This comes with the acknowledgement that often the best option is trying to avoid the court system altogether (see Chapter 13).

Navigating the Family Court System

The family court system is designed to manage a variety of family-related matters, including those involving PA. Understanding how the system works and what to expect can be helpful when dealing with such a challenging issue. Here are some key steps to take when navigating the family court system:

- Familiarise Yourself with the Process: In addition to Chapter 15, take the time to learn about the family court system in your jurisdiction and the specific procedures for handling child custody and access disputes. Understanding the process can help you better advocate for your child's best interests and prepare for court proceedings.
- File an application: If you suspect that PA is occurring and it is affecting your child's wellbeing, you may need to file an application with the family court for a child arrangement order or a modification of an existing order. This application should outline your concerns and provide evidence of the alienating behaviours, if possible.
- Attend Court Hearings: Be prepared to attend court hearings and actively participate in the process. During these hearings, you may have the opportunity to present evidence, call witnesses, and make arguments in support of your position.
- Comply with Court Orders and Directions: Throughout the process, it is crucial to comply with any court orders or directions. This may include attending mediation, participating in a parenting education program, or cooperating with a court-appointed expert for a custody evaluation.
- Stay Focused on Your Child's Best Interests: When navigating the family court system, always keep your child's best interests at the forefront of your decision-making. Be prepared to compromise and work cooperatively with the other parent, if possible, to achieve a resolution that is in the best interest of your child.

Obtaining Legal Representation

Having an experienced family lawyer on your side can be invaluable when dealing with PA. Here are some tips for finding and working with a legal representative:

- Research and Referrals: Start by researching family lawyers or solicitors in your area who have experience with PA cases, also sometimes known as high-conflict, hostile or intractable or complex cases. Consult with friends, family members, or support group members who have dealt with similar issues for recommendations.
- Initial Consultation: Schedule an initial consultation with potential lawyer to discuss your case and assess their level of expertise, experience, and approach to handling PA cases. This consultation is an opportunity to ask questions, share your concerns, and determine if the attorney is a good fit for your needs.
- Establish Clear Lines of Communication: Once you have retained a lawyer, establish a clear line of communication, and make sure you understand their preferred method of contact. Keep your lawyer informed about any developments in your case and promptly respond to their requests for information or documentation.
- Be Prepared to Share Information: Provide your attorney with all relevant information and documentation related to your case, including a history of the relationship with the other parent, any incidents of alienating behaviour, and evidence of your involvement in your child's life.
- Trust Your Lawyer's Expertise: While it is important to be informed and involved in your case, remember that your attorney is an experienced professional who is there to guide you through the process. Trust their expertise and be open to their advice and recommendations. But also feel free to respectfully challenge them if you think they haven't quite got something right.

PREPARING FOR COURT PROCEEDINGS

Preparing for court proceedings can be a stressful and overwhelming experience, but proper preparation is essential for presenting a convincing case. Here are some tips for preparing for court proceedings in PA cases:

- Organise Your Documentation: Gather and organise all relevant documentation related to your case, including records of communication with the other parent, evidence of the alienating behaviours, and any reports or evaluations from mental health professionals or other experts. Having a well-organised file can help you present a clear and coherent case to the court.

- Develop a Timeline: Create a detailed timeline of events, including significant milestones in your relationship with the other parent, incidents of alienating behaviour, and any actions you have taken to address the issue. This timeline can be a useful tool for presenting your case and demonstrating the progression of the alienation.
- Prepare for Cross-Examination: In court, you may be cross-examined by the other party's lawyer. Work with your lawyer to anticipate potential questions and prepare thoughtful, concise responses. Be honest and avoid becoming defensive or argumentative.
- Practice Testimony: If you are called to give evidence, practice delivering your testimony in a clear, calm, and well-organised manner. Your lawyer can help you refine your testimony and ensure that you are prepared to effectively communicate your concerns and experiences to the court.
- Identify and Prepare Witnesses: If you have witnesses who can provide relevant testimony, such as family members, friends, or professionals who have observed the alienating behaviours or their impact on your child, work with your lawyer to prepare them for their testimony. Ensure that they understand the purpose of their testimony and the importance of being truthful and objective.
- Dress Appropriately and Maintain Professionalism: On the day of the court hearing, dress professionally and conservatively. Be punctual and respectful and maintain a calm demeanour throughout the proceedings. Your conduct in court can have an impact on the judge's impression of you and the credibility of your case.

Successfully Managing the Court Process

Successfully managing the court process involves more than just preparing for court hearings. It also means understanding the dynamics of the court, maintaining a child-focused approach, and effectively communicating with all parties involved. Here are some strategies for managing the court process:

- Understanding Court Dynamics: The dynamics of the court can greatly influence the outcome of your case. It is essential to understand the role of the judge, the lawyers, and the child welfare experts involved in your case. This includes understanding their perspectives, their decision-making processes, and the factors they consider important in child custody cases.
- Maintaining a Child-focused Approach: Throughout the court process, keep your focus on the best interests of your child. Avoid personal attacks against the other parent and instead focus on the specific behaviours that are causing harm to your child. Demonstrate your commitment to promoting your child's wellbeing and maintaining their relationship with both parents where safe and appropriate.

- Effective Communication: Effective communication is crucial in managing the court process. This includes clear communication with your lawyer, with the other parent (if possible and appropriate), and with the court. Be honest, consistent, and concise in your communication. Avoid emotional language and focus on the facts.
- Managing Your Emotions: Court proceedings can be emotionally charged, especially in cases of PA. It is crucial to manage your emotions effectively both inside and outside the courtroom. This might mean seeking support from a counsellor or therapist, practising stress management techniques, or joining a support group for alienated parents.
- Adhering to Court Orders: Compliance with all court orders is crucial. Even if you disagree with a court order, it is important to adhere to it while you seek legal advice on your next steps. Non-compliance can negatively impact the court's perception of you and could have consequences for your case.
- Continuous Documentation: Throughout the court process, continue documenting instances of PA, your interactions with the child, and any communication with the other parent. This documentation can provide valuable evidence if your case returns to court.
- Seeking Expertise: Consider consulting with experts in PA, such as psychologists or therapists, who can provide reports or testimony to support your case. Their professional insights can be instrumental in helping the court understand the dynamics of PA.
- Addressing Potential Bias: Court processes are designed to be fair and impartial, but biases may sometimes emerge unintentionally. Traditional societal roles can occasionally influence the court's perception, leading to an unconscious bias towards one parent. Be aware of this and ensure that your lawyer understands and is prepared to address any potential biases. It's essential that you maintain your professionalism, present your case based on the child's best interests, and offer evidence to counter any misconceptions or stereotypes. This will ensure the focus stays on the facts of the case and the child's welfare.
- Preparing for the Long Haul: Court cases involving PA can take a long time to resolve, often involving many court appearances over months or even years. Prepare yourself for this reality both emotionally and practically. Ensure you have the support systems in place to help you cope with the long-term nature of these proceedings.
- Prioritising Mental Health: The court process in cases of PA can be incredibly stressful and may take a toll on your mental health. It is essential to prioritise self-care and mental wellness throughout this process. This may mean seeking support from a mental health professional, leaning on your support network of family and friends, or using stress management techniques such as mindfulness, exercise, or journaling. By taking care of your mental health, you are better equipped to navigate the court process and advocate for your child's best interests. Remember,

seeking help is a sign of strength, not weakness, and there are many resources available to support you in this journey.

Dealing with Disappointing Outcomes and Ongoing Lack of Contact

Despite your best efforts, there may be instances where the court's decision does not favour your desired outcome. It can be incredibly disheartening and even devastating, particularly when it results in an ongoing lack of contact with your child. However, it is crucial to remember that this is not the end of the road, and there are still steps you can take to maintain a connection with your child and work towards a better outcome.

- Seek Legal Counsel: If the court's decision is not in your favour, consult with your lawyer about potential options. This may include filing for an appeal, requesting a review, or considering other legal avenues.
- Maintain a Positive Outlook: Though it's natural to feel negative emotions, try to maintain a positive outlook for both your own mental health and your child's. Remember, court decisions can be subject to change, and the situation can improve over time.
- Keep Trying to Connect: Even if contact is limited, continue making efforts to connect with your child. This could involve sending letters, emails, gifts, or simply making sure your child knows you are always there for them.
- Keep Records: Keep a record of all your attempts to connect with your child. This can be used as evidence of your ongoing commitment to your child's life if you return to court.
- Self-Care: It is essential to take care of your physical and mental health during this challenging time. Reach out to support groups, talk to a therapist, maintain a healthy lifestyle, and engage in activities that help you cope with stress.
- Continue Educating Yourself: Stay informed about PA and potential strategies for dealing with it. Knowledge can empower you and give you hope.
- Seek Support: Connect with support groups or other individuals who have been through similar situations. Their experiences, advice, and support can be invaluable.
- Stay Hopeful: Many alienated parents eventually reconnect with their children. As your child grows and matures, they may seek to understand and reconnect. Be patient and keep the door open for them.

Self-Representation

The prospect of navigating the family court system can be daunting, especially for parents who are unable to afford a lawyer. However, it is important to know that you can represent yourself in court, a process known as "litigating in person" or self-representation.

- Understand Your Rights and Responsibilities: When you choose to represent yourself, you take on all the responsibilities that a solicitor would typically handle. This includes preparing your case, filing documents, presenting your argument, and adhering to legal procedures and court etiquette. You'll also be held to the same standards as a solicitor when it comes to knowing and understanding the law.
- Learn About the Legal Process: Invest time in understanding the UK's family court system and processes. This includes learning about the different stages of court proceedings, the specific laws that apply to your case, the court rules, and the paperwork that needs to be completed.
- Use Available Resources: Several resources are available to assist litigants in person. You can find detailed guides and resources for self-representing individuals at the Citizens Advice Bureau and the Advicenow website. Court staff can also provide procedural advice, but remember, they cannot provide you with legal advice.
- Court Forms and Documentation: It is crucial to familiarise yourself with the court forms and documents you will need. These will need to be filled out correctly and submitted on time. Misunderstandings or mistakes can cause delays in your case or negatively impact your case.
- Prepare Your Case: Organise all your evidence, create a timeline of events, and note down the main points you want to communicate to the court. Practice how you will present your case, keeping your language simple and focusing on the facts.
- Remain Professional: It is important to remain calm, polite, and professional throughout the court process. Listen carefully, address the judge as "Your Honour," and ensure that your questions and comments are respectful and relevant.

Remember, self-representation requires substantial effort and preparation. If it's an option, consult with a solicitor at least once to understand the specifics of your case better and ensure you're on the right track. It may also be worth reaching out to organisations and firms to see if they are able to help conduct the work on a "pro-bono" basis.

International Custody Disputes

International custody disputes can add an extra layer of complexity to PA cases. These disputes arise when parents live in different countries, or when one parent moves the child across international borders without the other parent's consent.

- Understand the Hague Convention: The Hague Convention on the Civil Aspects of International Child Abduction is an international treaty that provides a legal framework for resolving international child abduction cases, including some custody disputes. The UK is a signatory to this Convention. If your case is within the scope of this Convention, it can help ensure the prompt return of the child to their country of habitual residence.
- Legal Assistance: These cases can be legally complex due to the involvement of different legal systems. Retaining a lawyer who has experience in international family law can be extremely beneficial.
- Contact Reunite International: Reunite International Child Abduction Centre is a UK-based charity offering advice, information, and support to parents involved in international child abduction cases.
- Cooperate with Central Authorities: Each country that is a signatory to the Hague Convention has a Central Authority designed to help parents in these situations. In the UK, the Central Authority is part of the Official Solicitor's Department.
- Document Everything: Keep records of all communications and actions related to your case. This could be crucial evidence to support your case in court.
- Emotional Support: The emotional toll of an international custody dispute can be heavy. Seek support from professionals, family, friends, and support groups to help you through this challenging time.

ADVICE FOR CHILDREN INVOLVED IN LEGAL PROCEEDINGS (WRITTEN FOR KIDS)

Being involved in family court can feel confusing, scary, or even unfair. You may feel like you are caught in the middle of your parents' arguments or that you are being asked to make choices no child should have to make. These feelings are normal, and it is important to know that what is happening is not your fault. Courts, judges, and professionals are there to try to make decisions that help keep you safe and supported.

Understanding What's Happening

When families cannot agree on living arrangements or contact, the court sometimes has to step in. This does not mean anyone has "won" or "lost." Instead, the court's job is to think carefully about what will be best for you in the long run. Judges and professionals may ask questions about your life, your feelings, and your routines so they can understand what matters most to you.

Sharing Your Voice Safely

Your views are important, and adults involved in your case should take them seriously. At the same time, it can feel hard to know what to say if you feel pressured or worried about upsetting one of your parents. Remember:

- You are allowed to have your own thoughts and feelings.
- It is okay to feel love for both parents, even if they do not get along.
- If you are worried or confused, you can tell a trusted adult (such as a guardian ad litem, social worker, or therapist) who will make sure your feelings are heard in the right way.

You never have to take sides. The court is there to help you have safe, healthy relationships and to protect you if something is wrong.

Looking After Yourself

Court cases can take a long time, and during this time, you might feel stressed, angry, or sad. Some things that might help include:

- Talking to someone you trust, like a grandparent, teacher, or counsellor, about how you feel.
- Keeping a private journal or drawing your thoughts if you find it hard to talk.
- Doing activities you enjoy, sports, music, games, or spending time with friends, to give yourself a break from the stress.
- Reminding yourself that the problems between your parents are not your fault, even if it sometimes feels that way.

Hope for the Future

Sometimes, family situations can feel like they will never get better. But many children find that, as time passes, things become easier and relationships can heal. Courts, counsellors, and other adults are there to help make sure that you can grow up feeling safe, supported, and loved.

Remember: you are not responsible for fixing your parents' disagreements. Your job is to be a child. The adults, including the court, are responsible for making the big decisions. What matters most is that you are cared for, listened to, and able to look forward to your future.

ADVICE FOR LEGAL PROFESSIONALS

Family court professionals play a decisive role in cases involving PA. For alienated parents, court is often their only remaining avenue for restoring or protecting their relationship with their child. Many of these parents describe feeling unheard, misunderstood, or even vilified in proceedings. The following advice reflects what alienated parents consistently wish professionals understood when managing these complex and emotionally charged cases.

Take Allegations of PA Seriously

Alienated parents want you to know that PA is not simply a matter of "high-conflict parenting." It is a form of psychological harm that can fundamentally damage a child's development and sever their relationship with a loving parent. When parents raise concerns about alienation, they are usually not doing so to "win" a case, but because they are desperate to preserve their bond with their child. Listen carefully, look for patterns, and avoid dismissing PA as tactical or exaggerated without thorough assessment.

Avoid Gendered Assumptions

Alienated parents are acutely aware of how gender stereotypes influence court decisions. Fathers often fear being dismissed as less nurturing or inherently dangerous; mothers sometimes feel accused of alienation when raising legitimate concerns about abuse. Both experiences point to the same problem: bias undermines fairness. Approach each case on its evidence rather than on assumptions about what fathers or mothers "typically" do.

Ensure the Child's Voice is Contextualised

Parents want professionals to respect their child's voice, but also to understand how easily it can be influenced. An alienated child may sound certain and convincing in rejecting one parent, but this certainty can be the product of sustained manipulation. Alienated parents hope that legal professionals will listen to their children with compassion while also asking: *what might be shaping these views?*

Work with Competent Experts

Parents consistently emphasise the importance of expert input, but only when the experts are properly qualified. They fear that poorly trained or biased evaluators will misinterpret the dynamics at play and inadvertently entrench the alienation. They want legal professionals to ensure that any expert testimony or evaluations come from individuals with genuine expertise in PA, family systems, and trauma, and to scrutinise unsupported or unregulated claims to expertise.

Act Swiftly and Decisively

For alienated parents, time is critical. Every month that passes without meaningful contact deepens the rupture and makes reunification more difficult. Delays in proceedings or weak enforcement of orders can be devastating. Parents want legal professionals to treat PA cases with urgency, ensuring that court directions are followed promptly and consequences for non-compliance are clear.

Maintain a Child-Centred, Trauma-Informed Focus

Above all, alienated parents want professionals to remember that their children are the ones most affected. They ask that judges, lawyers, and evaluators approach cases with empathy, informed by the psychological realities of alienation. This means seeing beyond the adversarial battle between parents and keeping the long-term wellbeing of the child at the centre of every decision.

SUMMARY

This chapter has offered tailored guidance for parents, children, and legal professionals navigating the complex and emotionally taxing realities of PA within legal proceedings. For parents, advice focused on understanding the court process, securing effective representation, preparing evidence, and maintaining resilience through what is often a lengthy and exhausting journey. Children were provided with age-appropriate reassurance and strategies for expressing their feelings safely, protecting their wellbeing, and remembering that the conflict between parents is not their responsibility. For legal professionals, the chapter conveyed what alienated parents most want them to hear: to treat PA seriously, avoid bias, contextualise the child's voice, ensure expert testimony is credible, and act with urgency.

Taken together, these perspectives underline the immense strain placed on families in PA cases while pointing towards constructive strategies for support. By equipping parents, children, and professionals with practical tools and insights, the chapter emphasises that even within a difficult legal framework, there are ways to protect children's long-term wellbeing, sustain hope for healthier family relationships, and move closer to fairer, more child-centred outcomes.

BIBLIOGRAPHY

Cross, R., & Jagannmohan, M. (2021). *A practical guide to practice direction 12J and domestic abuse in private law children proceedings*. Law Brief Publishing.

Jordan, D. (2021). *How to divorce a narcissist: And succeed in the family court*. Independently Published.

Joshi, A. S. (2022). *Litigating parental alienation: Evaluating and presenting an effective case in court*. American Bar Association.

King, S., & Shama, F. (2022). *A practical guide to parental alienation in private and public law children cases*. Law Brief Publishing.

Lorandos, D., & Bernet, W. (Eds.). (2020). *Parental alienation: Science and law*. Charles C Thomas Publisher, Ltd.

McKenzie Friends Hub. (2025). *Navigating family court: A McKenzie friends guide*. McKenzie Friends Hub.

Reed, L. (2022). *The family court without a lawyer: A handbook for litigants in person* (4th ed.). Bath Publishing.

Rice, A. (2024). *Navigating family court with a high conflict person*. Independently Published.

17

INTERVENTION AND TREATMENT

If PA has been clearly identified then the next critical step is intervention. The damage caused by such relational disruption is not only psychological but often structural, fracturing family systems and distorting foundational attachments. Accordingly, therapeutic efforts aimed at restoring the child's bond with the alienated parent must be deliberate, evidence-informed, and sensitive to the complex trauma experienced by all parties involved.

This chapter explores a range of treatment and reunification approaches, focusing on what is currently known about their efficacy, limitations, and applicability in real-world contexts. Drawing on psychological, legal, and family systems perspectives, it provides guidance for professionals and families seeking to repair disrupted relationships. Interventions are framed not simply as therapeutic modalities but as relational processes embedded within broader socio-legal systems that must also be addressed to facilitate sustainable healing.

While there is no one-size-fits-all solution, a growing body of empirical evidence, alongside clinical practice and lived experience, has begun to illuminate what works, for whom, and under what conditions. The aim here is not only to evaluate these approaches but to consider how they might be embedded within coordinated systems of care, offering hope for families navigating the long shadow of alienation.

DOI: 10.4324/9781003630944-22

THERAPEUTIC INTERVENTIONS: MATCHING APPROACH TO CONTEXT

Intervening in cases of parental alienation requires nuanced, context-sensitive application of therapeutic modalities. No single intervention will work in every case; rather, the efficacy of any approach depends not only on the degree of alienation but also on the profile of the alienating parent and the specific dynamics at play within the family. In this section, three central therapeutic modalities are discussed, family therapy, individual therapy, and reunification therapy, each with its unique scope, limitations, and appropriateness depending on the stage of alienation and the behavioural patterns of the alienating parent.

Family Therapy

Family therapy can be effective in early to moderate stages of alienation, particularly when the alienating behaviours are less entrenched, or when both parents are willing to engage in a shared therapeutic space. It is particularly suited to loyalty conflicts or hybrid cases, where both parents may have contributed to a high-conflict dynamic, and the child's rejection is not yet rigid or psychologically embedded.

This modality is most effective when:

- The alienating parent is amenable to self-reflection and open to change, including acknowledgment of their role in the breakdown of family dynamics.
- Children remain in contact with both parents, even if this contact is strained or sporadic.
- The court or external authority can mandate and monitor engagement to ensure compliance and reduce manipulative sabotage of the process.

Family therapy is typically contraindicated in cases where the alienating parent engages in malignant narcissism, deliberate coercive control, or ongoing characterological enmeshment with the child, as these dynamics can contaminate the therapeutic space and reinforce harm rather than reduce it. In such cases, separate modalities, or court-ordered interventions, may be more appropriate.

Individual Therapy

Individual therapy is a foundational tool across all stages of alienation. It can be delivered to children, targeted parents, or (in rare cases where feasible) alienating parents. Its strength lies in offering a private, safe therapeutic alliance where complex emotions, identity disruptions, and trauma responses can be addressed without external pressures.

For children, individual therapy is particularly useful when:

- They are beginning to show ambivalence rather than complete rejection, suggesting some internal conflict or awareness of the distortion.
- There is evidence of induced anxiety, self-blame, or splitting in their internal representations of parents.
- The child is capable of forming a therapeutic alliance independent of the alienating parent's influence.

For targeted parents, individual therapy serves to:

- Rebuild identity and resilience after prolonged character assassination, institutional betrayal, and relational trauma.
- Develop coping strategies for navigating systems that may inadvertently perpetuate alienation (e.g., legal and social services).
- Prevent the transgenerational transmission of trauma by strengthening the parent's capacity to engage, when appropriate, in reunification efforts with attuned empathy rather than defensive reactivity.

Individual therapy for alienating parents is rare and often unsuccessful unless the parent is motivated for genuine change and able to acknowledge harm. In cases of high-conflict personality structures or coercive enmeshment, individual therapy may be resisted or subverted, and careful risk-benefit analysis is warranted.

Reunification Therapy

Reunification therapy is a highly specialised and often court-mandated intervention aimed at restoring the parent–child bond in moderate to severe cases of alienation. However, its appropriateness is highly contingent on case specifics, including:

- The extent of the alienation (e.g., complete rejection versus intermittent withdrawal).
- The risk posed by the alienating parent, including ongoing manipulation or sabotage.
- The capacity of the child to engage in emotionally demanding relational work.

Reunification therapy is most effective when:

- The child demonstrates ambivalence rather than hatred, and some memory or evidence of a prior secure bond remains.
- There is external support or containment (e.g., court orders, therapeutic supervision, or neutral placement).

- The intervention is part of a broader ecosystem of care, including therapeutic oversight, legal monitoring, and parent coaching.

This approach becomes risk-laden or even harmful when:

- The child has been subject to intense psychological splitting, rendering them unable to tolerate proximity to the targeted parent without dysregulation.
- The alienating parent maintains primary control over the child's environment, and undermines the process covertly or overtly.
- The therapy is applied prematurely or without adequate preparation, potentially retraumatising the child or reinforcing narratives of victimisation.

In such cases, pre-reunification work, including psychoeducation, systems intervention, and sometimes even temporary separation from the alienating environment, may be required before reunification can be ethically or effectively attempted.

THE EFFICACY AND LIMITATIONS OF INTERVENTION APPROACHES

The therapeutic imperative to intervene in cases of PA is widely recognised, particularly when the behaviours involved rise to the level of psychological abuse. However, the pathway to effective intervention is complex, contested, and, at times, fraught with ethical, legal, and clinical dilemmas. Nowhere is this more evident than in debates around reunification therapy and structured residential programmes, which have become focal points for both advocacy and critique.

The Case for Intervention

A growing body of literature and practice-based evidence supports the notion that specialist interventions can successfully repair alienated relationships, especially when implemented early and tailored to family-specific dynamics. Some studies suggest that modifying custodial arrangements, such as transferring residence to the targeted parent, can reduce exposure to alienating behaviours and facilitate emotional reconnection. Similarly, specialised family therapy and coordinated judicial-therapeutic approaches, where legal and clinical professionals collaborate with a shared understanding of alienation dynamics, have shown promise in restoring contact and ameliorating harm.

These interventions are often justified on the basis that parental alienation is a form of emotional abuse, and that failure to act perpetuates significant developmental, relational, and psychological harm to the child. Where the rejection of a previously loved parent cannot be explained by abuse, neglect, or demonstrably poor parenting, the ethical imperative becomes clear: the child's rejection is not a free expression of autonomy but the outcome of coercive manipulation and distorted attachment narratives. In these contexts, therapeutic and legal intervention is not only justified but necessary to uphold the child's right to a meaningful relationship with both parents.

Controversies and Challenges

Despite this rationale, serious questions remain about the robustness, safety, and empirical foundation of many current intervention models, particularly intensive reunification programmes, some of which involve temporary child removal or immersion in residential therapeutic settings. While these interventions have gained popularity in parts of North America and Europe, the evidence base remains limited, often comprising small samples, inconsistent methodologies, and non-independent evaluations. Meta-analyses have highlighted concerns about selection bias, lack of control groups, and limited follow-up data, making it difficult to assess long-term efficacy or potential harms.

A central tension in this debate lies in risk-balancing: how to weigh the potential trauma of removing a child from the care of the alienating parent against the damage of leaving them embedded in an abusive relational dynamic. In some cases, courts have ordered a reversal of custody to remove children from psychologically harmful environments. While such decisions may ultimately lead to positive outcomes, they are not without risk of retraumatisation, especially if the child has been psychologically programmed to fear or hate the targeted parent. Without adequate preparation, containment, and post-transition support, such removals can amplify distress, damage the child's sense of safety, and further entrench rejection.

Moreover, many critics, especially those sceptical of PA as a concept, have argued that reunification therapies risk pathologising children's resistance without sufficient exploration of possible underlying trauma, including abuse or neglect. In rare but real cases, what is framed as alienation may in fact be a justified estrangement, and the therapeutic goal should not be reunification but protection. As such, differential diagnosis and forensic-level assessment are critical preconditions to any intrusive intervention.

RECOMMENDATIONS FOR EFFECTIVE INTERVENTION IN PARENTAL ALIENATION CASES

The treatment of PA must be approached not as a conventional family conflict issue but as a form of psychological abuse that demands a protective, child-focused, and evidence-informed response. The efficacy of interventions varies substantially depending on the severity of alienation, the psychological profile of the alienating parent, and the professional competencies of those delivering the intervention. Crucially, traditional approaches such as generic family therapy, mediation, or child-led contact decisions are contraindicated in many of these cases and may exacerbate the harm.

Core Principles of Effective Intervention

Despite the inherent challenges, many families do experience significant improvements in relational functioning when interventions are well-structured and appropriately matched to case dynamics. Four foundational principles guide the effective treatment of parental alienation:

1. *Early, Decisive Action*: Intervention is most effective when applied before the child's rejection becomes deeply entrenched. Early signs of loyalty conflicts or subtle alignment should prompt preventive measures to avoid psychological splitting and identity diffusion.
2. *Tailored Approach by Severity*: Intervention strategies must be graduated by severity – mild, moderate, or severe – rather than delivered through a one-size-fits-all model. Each severity level calls for specific clinical and legal responses that reflect the child's symptoms, parental behaviours, and systemic influences.
3. *Specialist Clinical Involvement*: Professionals involved in the treatment of PA must have specialist training in coercive control, high-conflict family dynamics, and attachment-based disruptions. Unskilled therapeutic engagement risks validating distorted beliefs, reinforcing overempowerment in the child, or colluding with alienating behaviours.
4. *Integrated Legal-Therapeutic Response*: The synchronisation of legal enforcement with therapeutic care is essential. Court orders, sanctions, parenting time enforcement, and therapist updates must function as a coherent system designed to contain abuse and facilitate healing.

Best Practices by Severity

Mild Alienation

In cases of mild alienation, where a child is reluctant but not rejecting, and the alienating behaviours are less pervasive, early psychoeducation and relational support can be effective. Recommended strategies include:

- Psychoeducational family counselling, with a focus on communication, parenting skills, and exposure to corrective experiences.
- Parenting time enforcement, ensuring that both parents have quality and uninterrupted contact.

- Parenting coordination, especially by professionals trained in PA, to monitor compliance, reduce conflict, and support behavioural change.
- Court orders requiring the alienating parent to cease undermining behaviours, often with explicit consequences for noncompliance.
- Clear behavioural expectations for children, particularly adolescents, regarding adherence to court-ordered schedules and respect for both parents.

Although mild cases are less severe, they are often early stages in a potentially escalating pattern. Interventions must be assertive enough to disrupt the emerging dynamics and prevent progression into moderate or severe alienation.

Moderate Alienation

When alienation progresses to a moderate level, marked by persistent rejection, entrenched narratives, and greater psychological splitting, intervention must intensify. Effective approaches include:

- Individual therapy for each family member, coordinated across professionals to avoid triangulation and manipulation. These must include:
  - Therapy for the alienating parent to address indoctrination and psychological control.
  - Therapy for the targeted parent to reduce reactivity and enhance attachment-focused parenting.
  - Therapy for the child, not as a stand-alone solution but as a space for processing conflict, with integration into broader family goals.
- Continued parenting coordination, now serving a more forensic role to document compliance or sabotage.
- Court-enforced behavioural constraints that may enhance the authority of the targeted parent (e.g., requiring their consent for child activities or educational decisions).
- Regular judicial oversight, with feedback loops from therapists and coordinators to ensure ongoing accountability.

Moderate cases require close monitoring, as alienating behaviours often continue covertly. Without enforcement or meaningful consequences, therapeutic gains are easily reversed.

Severe Alienation

Severe alienation is a child protection emergency, not a therapeutic challenge alone. At this stage, the child may adamantly refuse contact, harbour irrational fear or hatred, and demonstrate the full behavioural profile of alienation (see Chapter 4). The alienating parent typically presents with obsessive, controlling, and entrenched behaviours and often lacks insight.

In such cases, the following best practices apply:

- Swift custody reversal, removing the child from the influence of the alienating parent. This is often the only viable route to deconstructing the abuse pattern.
- Structured reunification programmes, such as *Family Bridges* or *Turning Points for Families*, which use empirically validated models to restore balanced perceptions and attachment bonds.
- Temporary no-contact orders (e.g., 90 days) for the alienating parent, adjusted based on behaviour and therapeutic readiness.
- Aftercare therapy for the alienating parent, including psychoeducation on the harm caused and structured pathways back to supervised contact.
- Gradual reintegration planning, managed by professionals and courts, with strict oversight and behavioural conditions attached.

Critically, in these cases, delays in intervention increase the likelihood of long-term psychological harm and identity diffusion in the child. Emerging research confirms that many children, post-reunification, report surprise and relief upon recognising the manipulation they were subjected to.

REJECTING HARMFUL AND INEFFECTIVE APPROACHES

Certain interventions, despite their popularity in general family therapy, are contraindicated in PA cases and should be avoided:

- *Prolonged child-led therapy* without parental involvement, which can validate distorted beliefs.
- *Uncoordinated individual therapy*, where multiple professionals work in silos, enabling manipulation and splitting.
- *Generic family therapy or mediation*, particularly when power is asymmetrical or coercive control is present.
- *Deference to the child's stated preferences* without recognising the potential for guilt-free hostility or psychological manipulation.

These models fail to address the relational cause of the alienation and instead risk exacerbating it.

SUMMARY

Parental alienation must be recognised and treated as a form of psychological abuse, requiring responses equivalent in seriousness and structure to other forms of child maltreatment. Effective intervention demands early identification, tiered therapeutic strategies matched to the severity of alienation, and a coordinated legal and clinical framework that prioritises child protection. In moderate to severe cases, spontaneous reunification is exceedingly rare, and failure to intervene can result in profound, lasting harm.

Yet, the landscape of intervention remains fraught with controversy. Reunification therapies, while potentially transformative, must be applied with ethical caution, empirical grounding, and clear clinical oversight. This chapter has called for a shift away from polarised positions and towards a model that is both rigorous and reflective, one that values evidence, contextual understanding, and the nuanced realities of each case.

To support alienated children and their families, we must move beyond generalised or ideologically driven approaches and embrace interventions that are specialised, accountable, and attuned to the complexities of coercive family dynamics. The ultimate goal is to protect children, rebuild severed relationships, and ensure that therapeutic and legal systems do more good than harm.

BIBLIOGRAPHY

Andreopoulos, E., & Wexler, A. (2022). The "solution" to parental alienation: A critique of the turning points and overcoming barriers reunification programs. *Journal of Family Trauma, Child Custody & Child Development*. https://doi.org/10.1080/26904586.2022.2049462

Avalle, D. S., Smith, B. J., Wiederman, M. W., & Garnica, C. B. (2022). How efficacious is building family bridges? What the legal and mental health fields should know about building family bridges and "parental alienation". *Journal of Family Trauma, Child Custody & Child Development*. https://doi.org/10.1080/26904586.2022.2066595

Barnett, A., & Riley, A. (2022). Experiences of parental alienation interventions. In J. Mercer & M. Drew (Eds.), *Challenging parental alienation: New directions for practitioners and parents*. Routledge.

Champion, K. M. (2022). Coercion in families and child resistance to contact with a parent after family separation. *Journal of Family Trauma, Child Custody & Child Development*, 19, 230–243. https://doi.org/10.1080/26904586.2022.2105273

Chester, S. (2022). Reunification, alienation or re-traumatization? Let's stat listening to the child. *Journal of Family Trauma, Child Custody & Child Development*, 19, 359–382. https://doi.org/10.1080/26904586.2021.1957059

Haines, J., Matthewson, M., & Turnbull, M. (2020). *Understanding and managing parental alienation: A guide to assessment and intervention*. Routledge.

Harman, J. J., Saunders, L., & Afifi, T. (2022). Evaluation of the turning points for families (TPFF) program for severely alienated children. *Journal of Family Therapy*, 44, 279–298. https://doi.org/10.1111/1467-6427.12366

Mercer, J. (2022a). Attachment issues and reunification of parents and children. *Journal of Family Trauma, Child Custody & Child Development*, 19, 320–339. https://doi.org/10.1080/26904586.2022.2080147

Mercer, J. (2022b). Reunification therapies for parental alienation: Tenets, empirical evidence, commonalities, and differences. *Journal of Family Trauma, Child Custody & Child Development*. https://doi.org/10.1080/26904586.2022.2080147

Reay, K. M. (2015). Family reflections: A promising therapeutic program designed to treat severely alienated children and their family system. *The American Journal of Family Therapy*, 43(2), 197–207. https://doi.org/10.1080/01926187.2015.1007769

Templer, K., Matthewson, M., Haines, J., & Cox, G. (2017). Recommendations for best practice in response to parental alienation: Findings from a systematic review. *Journal of Family Therapy*, *39*, 103–122. https://doi.org/10.1111/1467-6427.12137

Trane, S. T., Champion, K. M., & Hupp, S. D. A. (2022). Comparison of parental alienation treatments and evidence-based treatments for children and families. In J. Mercer & M. Drew (Eds.), *Challenging parental alienation: New directions for professionals and parents*. Routledge.

Warshak, R. (2010). Family bridges: Using insights from social science to reconnect parents and alienated children. *Family Court Review*, *48*, 48–80.

Warshak, R. (2019). Reclaiming parent-child relationships: Outcomes of family bridges with alienated children. *Journal of Divorce and Remarriage*, *60*, 645–667. https://doi.org/10.1080/10502556.2018.1529505

Warshak, R. (2020). Parental alienation: How to prevent, manage, and remedy it. In D. Lorandos & W. Bernet (Eds.), *Parental alienation: Science and law* (pp. 142–206). Charles C Thomas Publisher, Ltd.

18

ADVICE ON TREATMENT

Intervening in alienation is not only a clinical or legal task; it is a deeply personal, relational journey for all involved. This chapter offers tailored guidance for those most directly impacted: alienated parents striving to reconnect with their children, alienating parents who may be willing or required to change their behaviours, children caught in the crossfire of divided loyalties, and professionals tasked with facilitating healing under difficult and often adversarial conditions. This chapter thus aims to empower each group with practical strategies, realistic expectations, and a grounded understanding of the path to relational repair. While no advice can offer a guaranteed resolution, clear, compassionate, and context-aware support can make a critical difference in navigating the difficult terrain of intervention.

ADVICE FOR ALIENATED PARENTS DURING INTERVENTION

Engaging in reunification or therapeutic intervention after experiencing parental alienation can be emotionally overwhelming. Even when a structured process is in place, the child may remain resistant or hostile, especially in the early stages. Alienated parents must therefore approach intervention with emotional discipline, reflective insight, and relational patience. The process is rarely linear, and success often depends as much on the targeted parent's capacity to tolerate distress as on the child's readiness to reconnect.

DOI: 10.4324/9781003630944-23

Be Open and Reflective

Even when alienation is clearly present, there is often value in reflecting honestly on one's past behaviour, not as a cause of the alienation but as a demonstration of maturity and openness. Acknowledging relational ruptures or previous mistakes, even small ones, can disarm a child's defences and allow space for renewed connection.

- Express genuine openness to feedback from your child or the therapist without becoming defensive.
- Avoid justifying or litigating past events; focus instead on how you can show up differently moving forward.
- Modelling accountability, however small, can help counteract the narrative of rejection and foster trust.

Take It Slow

Rebuilding a relationship cannot be rushed. Children emerging from an enmeshed or alienated dynamic may feel intense loyalty binds, fear of retribution, or internal confusion. Targeted parents must pace their expectations and recognise that emotional repair unfolds over time.

- Resist the urge to push for emotional closeness or immediate affection.
- Allow space for ambivalence, silence, or even testing behaviours without interpreting them as rejection.
- Focus on creating safe, predictable, low-pressure interactions, especially in the early stages of contact.

Do Not Take Rejection Personally

One of the hardest challenges during intervention is withstanding continued rejection or coldness from the child. However, these responses often reflect learned patterns rather than true emotional beliefs. Taking them personally or responding defensively can reinforce the alienating script.

- Understand that rejection may persist even after therapy begins; this does not mean the intervention is failing.
- Maintain emotional neutrality and show consistent warmth, even in the face of anger or disinterest.
- Remind yourself that the child's behaviour is often protective, not malicious.

Align with the Therapeutic Process

Interventions require collaboration. Therapists and coordinators must see the targeted parent as a reliable, emotionally regulated, and therapeutically engaged party. Building this perception can influence both the outcome and the professional narrative around the case.

- Attend sessions reliably, follow therapeutic guidance, and demonstrate flexibility.
- Avoid venting frustrations in the presence of the child or undermining the process through parallel communication.
- Communicate respectfully and constructively with professionals, even when decisions feel unfair or progress is slow.

Avoid Retaliation or Counter-Rejection

Even when hurt, alienated parents must avoid mirroring the alienation by withdrawing emotionally or retaliating when the child resists. While it may feel protective to "give up," doing so can confirm the child's belief that the relationship is broken or unsafe.

- Stay available and consistent, even when the child is inconsistent.
- Focus on long-term reconnection rather than short-term validation.
- Never speak negatively about the alienating parent to the child, even when their influence is evident.

Maintain Hope; But Stay Realistic

Intervention is a process of incremental change. Relationships often heal not through dramatic breakthroughs but through repeated, consistent, low-conflict experiences of safety and acceptance. Parents must hold hope while also preparing for slow progress, setbacks, and moments of emotional ambiguity.

- Celebrate small signs of openness, a shared activity, eye contact, a brief laugh, as signs of progress.
- Understand that resistance may flare at key milestones (e.g., holidays, transitions), and plan accordingly.
- Trust that secure attachment, once reactivated, can rebuild even after long periods of alienation.

ADVICE FOR ALIENATING PARENTS DURING INTERVENTION

Alienating parents are not a monolithic group. While some may engage in alienating behaviours deliberately and persistently, others may do so inadvertently, as a response to unresolved trauma, relational breakdown, or a distorted sense of protection. In cases where an alienating parent is mandated to participate in intervention, or expresses genuine willingness to support the child's relationship with the other parent, the therapeutic process presents both a challenge and an opportunity. The success of intervention often depends on the alienating parent's capacity for self-reflection, behavioural restraint, and commitment to the child's right to a relationship with both parents.

Acknowledge the Role You Have Played

The first, and often most difficult, step for many alienating parents is acknowledging that their own behaviours may have contributed to the child's rejection of the other parent. This does not require taking full blame or disregarding your own concerns, but it does mean recognising the impact of your actions, directly or indirectly, on the child's relational perceptions.

- Reflect on whether you have spoken negatively about the other parent, conveyed subtle disapproval, or rewarded rejection.
- Be open to feedback from professionals about your role, even when it is hard to hear.
- Acknowledgement is not weakness; it is a strength that signals readiness for change.

Prioritise the Child's Needs Over Your Own Emotions

Alienating behaviours often stem from strong emotions: hurt, betrayal, fear, or unresolved anger. These feelings are valid, but they must be managed separately from parenting decisions. The child's well-being, including their right to maintain loving bonds with both parents, must take precedence.

- Do not involve the child in adult disputes or use them as an emotional confidant.
- Avoid framing loyalty as a moral obligation or aligning love with rejection of the other parent.
- Ask yourself continuously: "Is this action serving my child's needs, or my own emotional state?"

Respect and Support the Therapeutic Process

Some alienating parents enter intervention reluctantly, often under court order. Others may express verbal support for reunification but subtly undermine the process. Regardless of initial stance, long-term outcomes improve when the alienating parent demonstrates genuine behavioural change and consistent support for the child's relationship with the other parent.

- Follow court orders and therapeutic recommendations, including parenting time schedules, without sabotage or passive resistance.

- Avoid coaching the child before sessions or interrogating them afterwards.
- Collaborate with professionals and take their concerns seriously, even when they challenge your perspective.

Avoid Defensive Narratives

It is common for alienating parents to feel misunderstood or misrepresented, especially in adversarial legal contexts. However, using the intervention space to defend or justify past actions can derail progress. The therapeutic focus must remain on the child's healing, not on vindicating one's own position.

- Avoid rehearsing grievances about the other parent in therapy or with the child.
- Focus instead on what the child needs now, and how you can contribute to a healthier dynamic going forward.
- Allow space for the child to form their own view of the other parent, without interference or distortion.

Prepare for Emotional Discomfort

Intervention can be emotionally threatening for alienating parents, particularly if they fear loss of control or retribution. It may also provoke intense anxiety as the child reconnects with the previously rejected parent. These responses are understandable, but must not be allowed to manifest in sabotage or renewed alienating behaviours.

- Seek individual therapy to explore and manage your own emotional reactions.
- Accept that the process may feel unfair or destabilising, but still necessary.
- Focus on your long-term relationship with the child, which is ultimately strengthened when both parental bonds are intact.

Commit to Change; Even if Reunification Feels Threatening

Some alienating parents fear being "replaced" or marginalised if the child reconnects with the targeted parent. This fear may drive renewed control attempts. But healthy attachment is not a zero-sum game. Children benefit from multiple secure relationships, and maintaining your role as a trusted caregiver requires letting go of relational gatekeeping.

- Reassure your child that it is safe and healthy to love both parents.
- Avoid testing the child's loyalty or interpreting affection for the other parent as a betrayal.
- Remember: the goal is not to win but to raise a well-adjusted child with full access to their family.

ADVICE FOR CHILDREN INVOLVED IN INTERVENTION

If you're a child or young person going through an intervention or therapy process because of problems between your parents, it can feel confusing, frustrating, or even scary. You might feel stuck in the middle, unsure who to trust, or torn between wanting to make people happy and needing space to figure out how you really feel. All of these feelings are completely normal. This section is for you, to help you understand what's happening and what might help as you move through this process.

It's Okay to Have Mixed Feelings

You might have been told or made to feel like one of your parents is unsafe, bad, or doesn't care about you. You might even believe that right now. But sometimes, when parents fight or say bad things about each other, it can make children feel like they have to take sides. This can cause confusion inside, like your heart and your head are saying different things.

- You don't have to sort out all your feelings right away.
- It's okay to feel close to one parent and unsure about the other.
- Feelings can change over time, and that's okay too.

You Are Not Responsible for Adult Problems

Whatever has happened between your parents, it is not your job to fix it, protect one of them, or carry the blame. Adults are supposed to take care of children, not the other way around. If a parent has said things that make you feel guilty, scared, or responsible, it's important to know that's not fair to you.

- You have the right to love both your parents, even if they don't get along.
- You're allowed to feel safe, free, and respected by both sides.
- This isn't your fault.

Give Yourself Time

Intervention or reunification doesn't mean everything has to go back to "normal" right away. It's okay if seeing or talking to a parent you've felt distant from feels weird or uncomfortable at first. You don't have to pretend, just be honest about where you're at, and take it one step at a time.

- You don't have to force hugs or conversations if it doesn't feel right.
- Sometimes just spending time together quietly is enough to start rebuilding things.
- Let things grow slowly. Trust comes back through experience, not pressure.

You Can Say What You Need, Respectfully

You might have strong opinions or concerns about your parents. That's okay. But it's important to share your thoughts respectfully, especially in therapy or when speaking to adults who are helping. Speaking up doesn't mean shouting or shutting people out, it means being honest, calm, and open.

- Try saying how you feel using "I" statements (e.g., "I feel nervous when . . .").
- If something feels wrong or uncomfortable, let the therapist or trusted adult know.
- Everyone involved in the intervention wants to help you feel safe.

Be Open to New Experiences

Sometimes, when you've gone a long time without seeing one parent, or you've only heard negative things, it can be hard to imagine that anything good could come from reconnecting. But people are often more complex than the stories we hear about them. Being open doesn't mean you have to forgive everything right away. It just means you're giving yourself a chance to learn and decide for yourself.

- Let yourself be curious, not just cautious.
- You're allowed to change your mind if new experiences feel different from what you expected.
- Remember, your thoughts and feelings belong to you, not anyone else.

You Deserve a Loving Relationship with Both Parents

Even if things have been difficult or messy, you have the right to have a relationship with both of your parents, as long as it's safe. Intervention is not about forcing you to do something you don't want. It's about helping you reconnect, in your own way, when the time is right, and with adults who support and protect you.

- A good parent wants what's best for you, even if that means letting you take your time.
- You don't have to choose between parents.
- You are deeply valued and loved, just for being you.

ADVICE FOR PROFESSIONALS SUPPORTING INTERVENTION

Professionals tasked with facilitating intervention in parental alienation cases, whether as therapists, evaluators, or parenting coordinators, operate in one of the most complex and emotionally fraught areas of practice.

Success often hinges not only on clinical skill but on systemic awareness, ethical clarity, and the ability to manage conflictual, high-stakes environments without losing sight of the child's best interests. This section provides practical guidance to support professionals in navigating this terrain with confidence and care.

Prioritise Child Protection Over Family Harmony

In alienation cases, the instinct to preserve family unity or avoid conflict can sometimes obscure the fact that one parent's behaviour may constitute psychological abuse. Professionals must remain vigilant to the power dynamics at play and resist applying standard models of shared responsibility when the evidence suggests coercive control.

- Be prepared to disrupt false equivalence; not all family conflict is mutual.
- Centre the child's right to safe and balanced relationships over any presumed need to "compromise."
- Avoid pressuring the child to forgive or reconcile on adult timelines; trust is earned, not imposed.

Avoid Generic Therapeutic Models

Standard family therapy or mediation approaches are often contraindicated in cases involving alienation. These can backfire when practitioners inadvertently validate distorted narratives, reinforce child overempowerment, or place alienated parents and alienating parents in the same moral frame.

- Use assessment tools and frameworks specific to PA and coercive dynamics.
- Maintain role clarity: reunification is not neutral ground; it involves recognising abuse and facilitating repair.
- Ensure interventions are trauma-informed, but also alienation-specific; these are not interchangeable concepts.

Stay Systemically Informed and Legally Aligned

Alienation cases often unfold across multiple systems, clinical, legal, educational, and professionals must work collaboratively across domains while maintaining clear boundaries.

- Communicate regularly with courts, coordinators, and other involved professionals.
- Keep records that are clear, factual, and ready to be used in forensic contexts if required.

- Understand the legal mandates shaping the case, but do not allow judicial deference to override your clinical judgement.

Maintain Emotional Neutrality and Relational Integrity

Professionals are often subject to intense pressure from both parents, as well as from emotionally distressed children. It is essential to remain calm, non-reactive, and boundary-aware, while still being warm, attuned, and emotionally available to all parties.

- Avoid being drawn into triangulation, rescuing, or covert alignment with either parent.
- Empathise with all family members, but do not confuse empathy with endorsement of harmful behaviours.
- Model the relational dynamics you hope to cultivate in the family: respect, regulation, and responsiveness.

Pace the Process and Prepare for Setbacks

Intervention in PA cases rarely follows a linear path. Children may regress, parents may sabotage, and systems may fail to enforce boundaries. Professionals must prepare families for this and avoid interpreting setbacks as therapeutic failure.

- Set realistic expectations from the outset and revisit them regularly.
- Frame early resistance as part of the process, not a sign of futility.
- Help families focus on process goals (e.g., improved communication, safe contact) rather than immediate outcomes.

Continue Professional Development

Given the evolving and contested nature of the PA field, professionals must commit to ongoing education and reflective practice. The difference between effective and harmful intervention often lies in training, supervision, and openness to complexity.

- Engage with peer-reviewed research and emerging best practices.
- Seek supervision, especially in ethically grey or emotionally charged situations.
- Be honest about the limits of your expertise, refer or collaborate when needed.

SUMMARY

Effective intervention in parental alienation requires not only structured therapeutic and legal strategies but also thoughtful engagement from each party involved. For alienated parents, this means approaching reunification with emotional restraint, openness, and a long-term mindset. For alienating parents, meaningful change begins with acknowledging their role and prioritising the child's right to balanced relationships. Children navigating intervention need reassurance, space to process mixed emotions, and protection from adult conflicts. Professionals, meanwhile, must apply alienation-specific models, maintain systemic awareness, and align clinical practice with child protection principles. By tailoring support to the unique needs and responsibilities of each group, interventions can become safer, more effective, and more ethically grounded.

19

THE ROLE OF BROADER SOCIETY

While parental alienation plays out within families, it does not arise, or persist, in a vacuum (as explored in Chapter 8). The attitudes, assumptions, and responses of wider society and its institutions can either challenge or enable alienating behaviours. From the way schools manage parental communication, to how the media frames high-conflict custody disputes, to the cultural norms that shape our understanding of parenting roles and post-separation families, societal structures profoundly influence the recognition and handling of PA. This chapter builds on the foundations laid in Chapter 8 by offering concrete recommendations for change across key domains: schools and educators, public discourse and media, cultural norms surrounding parenting and divorce, and broader policy frameworks. By examining the role of each, and identifying where reform is needed, we aim to show how a more informed, coordinated, and child-centred societal response can disrupt the enabling conditions of parental alienation and support healthier outcomes for affected families.

SCHOOLS AND TEACHERS: BUILDING INSTITUTIONAL CAPACITY TO RESPOND TO PARENTAL ALIENATION

Schools are often a child's most consistent environment during periods of familial instability. As such, they hold unique potential to either buffer the effects of parental alienation or, if poorly informed, reinforce alienating

DOI: 10.4324/9781003630944-24

dynamics through unintentional collusion or exclusion. To effectively protect and support children impacted by PA, schools must move beyond ad hoc responses and adopt a system-wide approach grounded in training, policy clarity, and inter-agency collaboration.

Training and Professional Development

All school personnel who interact with children, including teachers, pastoral leads, counsellors, and administrators, should receive specialised training on recognising and responding to the signs of parental alienation. This training should go beyond basic safeguarding and include:

- Recognising behavioural indicators of alienation, such as unexplained hostility towards one parent, sudden changes in effect, or rigid alignment with one parent's narrative.
- Understanding the psychological dynamics of alienation, including loyalty conflicts, psychological splitting, and enmeshment.
- Navigating communication with both parents, including how to maintain neutrality while ensuring that both legally recognised caregivers are informed and engaged.
- Avoiding unintentional collusion, such as removing one parent from communication loops or validating a child's rejection without appropriate clinical input.

Training should be integrated into existing safeguarding frameworks and repeated regularly to reinforce awareness and adapt to emerging research.

Policy Development and Safeguarding Integration

Clear, enforceable policies are essential for ensuring consistency in school responses to PA. These policies should be embedded within broader safeguarding and inclusion frameworks, and must address:

- Equal parental access to school communications and events unless explicitly restricted by a court order.
- Standard procedures for handling disputes between parents, including guidance on how and when to engage pastoral or safeguarding leads.
- Protocols for escalating concerns to social services or legal professionals when emotional harm is suspected.
- Confidentiality protections that balance the child's right to privacy with the duty of care owed to both parents.

Policy development should be done in consultation with legal, clinical, and safeguarding experts, and adapted to reflect local statutory requirements.

Implementation and Cultural Change

For policies and training to have a meaningful impact, schools must foster a culture of neutrality, compassion, and procedural integrity. This requires not just information dissemination but the active engagement of leadership teams in:

- Embedding training outcomes into school procedures and daily practices.
- Modelling non-partisan communication in interactions with parents.
- Appointing dedicated safeguarding or family liaison staff explicitly trained in high-conflict and alienation dynamics.

Whole-school implementation must also involve students, who should receive age-appropriate education on family diversity, healthy boundaries, and emotional regulation, creating a more informed and empathetic peer environment.

Inter-Agency Collaboration

Schools cannot manage PA alone. They must be empowered and expected to collaborate with external agencies, including:

- Child-welfare services, when emotional abuse or neglect is suspected.
- Mental health professionals, to facilitate access to therapeutic support for the child and, where appropriate, family systems.
- Parenting coordinators or family court services, when relevant, to provide input on contact compliance or behavioural observations.

Such collaborations should be formalised through clear referral pathways and confidentiality agreements, ensuring schools do not overstep their remit but are fully integrated into the protective network around the child.

GPS AND HEALTH SERVICES: CULTIVATING PROFESSIONAL CURIOSITY AND EARLY RECOGNITION

General practitioners (GPs), paediatricians, and allied health professionals often serve as the first point of contact for families in distress, making them uniquely positioned to identify early signs of parental alienation. However, without adequate training or awareness, these professionals may misinterpret the child's presentation, viewing alignment with one parent or rejection of the other as a natural response to separation, rather than a potential red flag.

To address this, health services must embed professional curiosity into their routine safeguarding and assessment practices. This involves:

- Asking deeper questions when a child presents with psychosomatic complaints, anxiety, or mood issues in the context of family separation.
- Observing patterns in which parent attends appointments, and whether the other parent is included or excluded from medical decisions without legal justification.
- Being alert to highly polarised narratives or adult language echoed by children in describing the other parent.
- Considering the possibility of emotional manipulation or coercive control when one parent consistently dominates health-related communication or access.

Health professionals should not attempt to resolve these dynamics themselves, but should be trained to document concerns carefully and refer families to appropriate safeguarding, legal, or mental health services. Inclusion of PA in standard child safeguarding training for all primary care and community health staff would represent a critical step forward in improving early intervention.

SOCIAL WORKERS AND CHILD PROTECTION PROFESSIONALS: RAISING STANDARDS OF ASSESSMENT AND ACTION

Social workers occupy a pivotal role in child safeguarding and welfare, yet many report feeling ill-equipped to assess or intervene in cases involving parental alienation. Traditional child protection frameworks often emphasise physical harm or neglect, while emotional abuse via psychological manipulation, especially when masked by a superficially "protective" parent, may go unrecognised or be inadvertently reinforced.

To address this, social work practice must evolve to meet the demands of complex family coercion dynamics, with a focus on:

Enhancing Training and Diagnostic Awareness

- Social workers must be trained to distinguish between alienation, estrangement, and justified rejection, using validated frameworks such as the five-factor model.
- Emotional abuse through alienation should be explicitly included in child protection guidelines, not left to individual interpretation.
- Training should include indicators of coercive control, overempowerment of the child, and the misuse of safeguarding claims.

Strengthening Professional Curiosity and Critical Evaluation

- Practitioners must avoid accepting the presenting parent's narrative at face value, especially when it is excessively negative or one-sided.

- Children who parrot adult language or show unwarranted fear, disdain, or cut-off behaviour towards one parent should trigger heightened scrutiny, not passive acceptance.
- Assessments must include observation of the child with both parents, not just interviews or reported accounts.

Accountability and Intervention

- Where alienation is identified, social workers must act decisively to protect the child's right to family connection, treating the alienating behaviour as a safeguarding concern.
- Reports to court must be balanced, evidence-based, and free from uncritical repetition of the child or alienating parent's account.
- Child protection agencies should develop clear protocols for responding to suspected PA, including when and how to escalate concerns or recommend specialist intervention.

By shifting practice from passive observation to active inquiry, and from surface-level neutrality to meaningful advocacy, social workers can play a decisive role in preventing the long-term emotional harm associated with parental alienation.

REFORMING THE FAMILY COURT SYSTEM: STRUCTURAL CHANGE FOR SYSTEMIC IMPACT

Despite increasing recognition of parental alienation within individual legal judgements, the family court system as a whole remains inconsistent, under-resourced, and often ill-suited to respond effectively to the complex dynamics of PA. Delays in proceedings, adversarial processes, limited enforcement mechanisms, and a lack of coordinated therapeutic support contribute to systemic inertia, leaving children exposed to ongoing emotional harm while protective interventions stall or falter. If the courts are to function as a true safeguard for alienated children, a fundamental shift in structure, culture, and resource allocation is required.

Prioritising Timeliness and Continuity

- Early identification and fast-tracking of high-conflict, alienation-risk cases is essential to prevent entrenchment. Long delays enable alienating dynamics to deepen and reduce the chances of successful intervention.
- Courts should assign consistent judicial oversight across the life of a case. Rotating judges or inconsistent rulings disrupt therapeutic continuity and undermine the authority of orders.

Embedding Specialisation and Multidisciplinary Expertise

- Courts need dedicated family judges and court teams with training in parental alienation, coercive control, and child psychological abuse.
- Wherever possible, proceedings should be informed by multidisciplinary panels, drawing on psychological, social work, and child development expertise to assess the best interests of the child holistically.

Replacing the Adversarial Model

- The traditional adversarial system, designed to determine winners and losers, is fundamentally at odds with the goal of restorative family justice. It incentivises positional arguments and punitive strategies, rather than cooperative problem-solving.
- Instead, courts should adopt a problem-solving, child-welfare orientation, with a focus on relational repair, structured intervention, and therapeutic oversight.

Strengthening Enforcement and Protective Powers

- One of the most critical weaknesses in current practice is the lack of enforcement when alienating parents breach court orders. This not only emboldens continued alienation but also undermines the court's credibility in the eyes of the child.
- Courts must have access to a graduated menu of enforceable responses, from parenting time enforcement to temporary custody changes and mandated therapeutic participation, all informed by a proportionality principle and centred on the child's long-term welfare.

Institutional Accountability and Evaluation

- Finally, systemic change requires transparency, data collection, and evaluative feedback. Courts should track outcomes in alienation-related cases, including the impact of custody decisions, enforcement actions, and reunification efforts.
- Ongoing audit, research, and oversight mechanisms should be implemented to ensure that decisions align with both clinical knowledge and children's developmental needs.

Until the family court system is reformed to recognise parental alienation not as a contested legal strategy but as a form of psychological abuse requiring coordinated response, children will continue to fall through the cracks of an inconsistent and often adversarial system.

MEDIA AND PUBLIC DISCOURSE: RESHAPING THE NARRATIVE AROUND PARENTAL ALIENATION

The media, both traditional and digital, plays a powerful role in shaping how society understands family conflict, divorce, and parent–child relationships. Yet when it comes to parental alienation, media coverage often veers towards simplistic narratives, reinforcing cultural stereotypes or sensationalising individual cases. At worst, this contributes to public confusion, judicial inconsistency, and professional hesitation to act, particularly when alienation is conflated with legitimate safeguarding concerns or gender-based violence.

If public discourse is to become part of the solution rather than part of the problem, media institutions must adopt a more responsible, nuanced, and child-centred approach.

Challenging Stereotypes and Polarised Frames

- Parental alienation is frequently misrepresented through gendered tropes, as either mothers being unjustly accused in the context of domestic abuse or fathers being vilified or erased from children's lives. Both framings obscure the core issue: the manipulation of a child to unjustifiably reject a once-loved parent, irrespective of gender.
- Journalistic coverage should resist binary or moralising narratives, and instead draw on the growing body of psychological and legal research that recognises alienation as a complex, context-sensitive form of emotional abuse.

Amplifying Accurate and Ethical Reporting

- Media outlets should develop editorial guidelines for reporting on high-conflict family law cases, including how to discuss PA without sensationalism or retraumatising affected children.
- Journalists should consult with clinical experts when reporting on cases involving alienation dynamics, just as they might consult medical experts when reporting on public health issues.
- Use of anonymous case summaries, informed by expert commentary, can help raise awareness while protecting privacy.

The Role of Social Media: Double-Edged Influence

- Social media platforms often serve as unregulated spaces where parental grievances are aired, sometimes in ways that expose or manipulate children, spread misinformation, or escalate family tensions.
- At the same time, social media can also amplify survivor voices, share accurate psychoeducational content, and provide communities of support for targeted parents and alienated children.

Recommendations for improving the digital ecosystem include:

- Encouraging platforms to adopt policies prohibiting the public sharing of content involving children in high-conflict custody disputes, particularly when it involves vilification of the other parent.
- Supporting content creators and influencers who share evidence-based, non-sensationalised information about parental alienation.
- Encouraging professional organisations, researchers, and advocacy groups to use social media to counter misinformation and promote informed discussion.

Shifting the Public Narrative

Ultimately, the media has the power to reshape public understanding of parental alienation; not as a fringe or fabricated issue but as a recognised form of psychological harm that can and should be addressed within legal, clinical, and societal frameworks. This requires moving beyond polarisation and towards compassionate accuracy, centred on the voices and long-term wellbeing of the children most affected.

CULTURAL NORMS AROUND SEPARATION AND DIVORCE: UNPACKING THE IDEOLOGICAL ROOTS OF PARENTAL ALIENATION

Parental alienation does not emerge solely from individual pathology or legal oversight; it is also a cultural phenomenon, sustained by entrenched societal beliefs about parenting, family breakdown, and post-separation roles. These cultural scripts can normalise exclusion, obscure emotional abuse, and foster environments in which children are subtly or overtly pressured to align with one parent against the other. To meaningfully prevent PA, we must address these underlying ideological conditions.

Idealised and Gendered Parent Roles

Many Western societies continue to uphold idealised, binary conceptions of motherhood and fatherhood. Mothers are frequently seen as primary, emotionally indispensable caregivers; fathers as peripheral, instrumental, or expendable. These stereotypes:

- Enable alienating behaviours by justifying exclusion as protection or necessity.
- Reinforce judicial hesitancy to enforce contact with non-resident parents, particularly fathers, even in the absence of safeguarding concerns.
- Diminish recognition of male victims of alienation and female perpetrators of coercive parenting.

A rebalancing is needed, one that recognises both mothers and fathers as equally capable of nurturing or harming, and that centres the child's right to meaningful relationships with both parents.

The Myth of "Children's Choices" in High-Conflict Contexts

Another prevailing cultural belief is that children, particularly adolescents, should be free to choose which parent they live with post-separation. While autonomy is important, this view:

- Ignores the developmental limitations of children in making fully informed decisions under duress, loyalty binds, or psychological manipulation.
- Places undue pressure on children to take sides, reinforcing splitting and emotional overempowerment.
- Obscures adult responsibility and masks coercion as "preference."

Public discourse must shift from treating children's expressed wishes as unassailable truth to interpreting them within developmental, emotional, and relational contexts, particularly when rejection appears disproportionate or inflexible.

Divorce as Disentanglement

Cultural narratives often frame divorce as a clean break; the severing of all ties, including emotional and relational ones. This notion, while perhaps emotionally useful for adults, is harmful when transposed onto the parent–child relationship. Unlike romantic ties, parenthood is lifelong and non-transferable.

This "clean break" mentality:

- Validates the exclusion of a parent as a legitimate form of boundary-setting or personal growth.
- Neglects the child's need for continuity of attachment, even in the face of parental conflict.
- Normalises relational cut-off as a reasonable coping strategy, rather than a red flag.

Cultural reframing is needed to reinforce the principle that parenthood endures beyond the end of a partnership, and that the child's identity and psychological stability often depend on access to both sides of their family.

What Cultural Change Requires

Addressing these discourses means engaging in public education, professional training, and media literacy campaigns that:

- Promote non-gendered understandings of caregiving and abuse.
- Teach the public and professionals to recognise emotional abuse and psychological manipulation, not just physical danger, as causes for concern.
- Challenge the idea that child resistance or preference is always evidence of autonomy, and not potentially a sign of distress or coercion.

Only through cultural shifts of this kind can we reduce the structural ambivalence that allows parental alienation to thrive in plain sight.

THE ROLE OF POLICYMAKING: LEGISLATIVE LEADERSHIP FOR CULTURAL AND SYSTEMIC CHANGE

No meaningful societal change around parental alienation can occur without strong, principled leadership at the level of policy. While clinicians, educators, and courts can intervene at the individual and institutional level, systemic prevention and redress require coordinated legislative action. Policymakers have a central role to play in setting the cultural tone, resourcing effective responses, and holding systems accountable to protect children's rights to safe, ongoing relationships with both parents.

Closing the Policy Gaps

Current legal and policy frameworks in many jurisdictions fail to adequately address the dynamics of PA. Inconsistent enforcement of court orders, lack of shared parenting presumptions, and weak recognition of emotional abuse leave significant space for alienating behaviours to flourish. Well-intended protective policies, such as those addressing domestic violence, can also be misapplied or weaponised, especially in systems that lack the tools to differentiate between genuine safeguarding concerns and coercively framed alienation strategies.

To close these gaps, policy reform must prioritise:

- Clear legal recognition of parental alienation as a form of psychological abuse, with an emphasis on its developmental harm to children.
- Integration of PA into domestic abuse frameworks, acknowledging that coercive control can be exercised through children, and that alienating behaviours often co-occur with patterns of intimate terrorism.
- Robust enforcement mechanisms for court-ordered parenting time, including graduated sanctions that are proportional, child-centred, and timely.
- A rebuttable presumption of shared parenting time (e.g., 50/50 care), which can shift the legal culture away from winner–loser dynamics and reduce opportunities for manipulation.

Criminalising Coercive Alienation

While controversial, the option of criminalising specific alienating behaviours, particularly when they amount to sustained psychological abuse, must be part of the policy conversation. Existing laws around coercive control, emotional abuse, and child endangerment could be extended or clarified to include alienation-related conduct. This would not mean criminalising parental conflict or imperfect co-parenting, but targeting intentional, sustained efforts to sever a child's bond with a loving parent through manipulation, false narratives, or obstruction of contact.

Evidence-Based, Interdisciplinary Policy Formation

Effective policy must be informed not only by legal precedent but also by clinical research, practitioner insight, and lived experience. A child-focused, evidence-driven approach would ensure that reforms are proportional, ethical, and grounded in developmental psychology. Policymakers must collaborate with psychologists, family law experts, educators, and those affected by PA to develop multi-sectoral responses that span health, education, welfare, and justice systems.

A Catalyst for Cultural Change

Ultimately, strong policy can serve as a cultural catalyst, sending a clear message that emotional abuse via parental alienation is not a private matter or unfortunate by-product of divorce, but a public issue requiring decisive action. Clear laws and frameworks not only guide practice but also shape public norms, helping to reframe how society understands post-separation parenting, children's rights, and the limits of adult autonomy in the family system.

In this way, policymakers are not just responding to the problem of parental alienation; they are redefining the social conditions in which it can no longer thrive.

SUMMARY

Parental alienation is sustained not only by individual behaviours and legal oversights, but by the broader societal and institutional contexts in which families exist. Schools, health services, social workers, and family courts all require specialised training, clear policies, and inter-agency collaboration to respond effectively. Meanwhile, the media and public discourse must move beyond sensationalism and polarised narratives to promote accurate, compassionate understanding. At the deepest level, cultural beliefs about parenting, divorce, and children's autonomy must be critically re-examined to prevent the normalisation of exclusion and psychological abuse. A coordinated, system-wide response, grounded in child protection principles and informed by evidence, is essential for dismantling the conditions that enable alienation and for promoting healthy, enduring relationships for children post-separation.

PART 5

WHAT CAN YOU DO ABOUT IT?

20

GENERAL ADVICE FOR TARGETED PARENTS

Parental alienation is often a prolonged, exhausting journey; marked by confusion, rejection, injustice, and, for many, profound grief. While earlier chapters have provided targeted advice for parents at specific stages of intervention or within particular institutional contexts, this chapter offers a broader roadmap. It is designed to support targeted parents across the full trajectory of alienation: from the early signs of misalignment, through the depths of estrangement, to potential recovery or reconnection. Rather than focusing solely on tactics, this chapter outlines core principles and strategies, emotional, legal, relational, and psychological, that can sustain parents through the unique challenges of this experience. Drawing on clinical evidence, expert consensus, and lived experience, it aims to help parents preserve their wellbeing, maintain hope, and act wisely in pursuit of protecting their child and restoring the relationship. While no path is the same, the principles outlined here can offer structure and strength amid the uncertainty.

PRACTICAL PRINCIPLES FOR TARGETED PARENTS

Parental alienation often unfolds over time and across systems. For targeted parents, the ability to act strategically, calmly, and consistently can make a vital difference; not only in preserving the possibility of reconnection, but

DOI: 10.4324/9781003630944-26

also in protecting your own mental health. This section outlines key practical principles to guide your approach throughout the alienation journey.

Communicating and Co-Parenting with a Difficult or Alienating Parent

Alienating parents often provoke conflict or escalate tensions in ways that can destabilise the child's relationship with the targeted parent. The goal is not to "win" these interactions but to avoid feeding the narrative of hostility and reinforce your credibility.

- Keep the child at the centre: Frame every communication around your child's needs, not your grievances.
- Stay factual and neutral: Use clear, unemotional language. Avoid blame or retaliation, even when provoked.
- Document all communication: Use written formats (texts, emails, parenting apps) and keep records.
- Use structured tools: Co-parenting apps can create boundaries, reduce ambiguity, and limit opportunities for manipulation.
- Avoid verbal altercations: Refuse to engage in in-person disputes. Calm disengagement is more powerful than reactive confrontation.

Building and Maintaining a Strong Support Network

Isolation is one of the greatest risks for targeted parents. Reconnection with your child often begins with connection elsewhere.

- Lean on trusted friends and family: Share openly with those who can support you without escalating conflict.
- Engage professionals early: Find therapists, legal advisors, and parenting coordinators experienced in PA.
- Join support groups: Connect with others who understand the dynamics of alienation. The validation and insight can be transformative.
- Educate yourself: Read widely on PA to build confidence, anticipate patterns, and recognise professional missteps.
- Stay visible in your child's life: Enlist allies, teachers, coaches, extended family, who can keep you anchored in your child's world.

Communicating with Alienated Children

Alienation changes how a child perceives you, but your role remains: to be the safe, loving, and available parent. Tailor your approach to the level of resistance.
Mild Alienation:

- Gently correct false beliefs without criticising the other parent.
- Create relaxed, pressure-free spaces for connection.
- Express love regularly, even when it's not returned.

Moderate Alienation:

- Persist calmly with contact, even if it's one-sided or rejected.
- Avoid over-apologising or begging; instead, convey confidence and openness.
- Work with a PA-informed therapist to manage sessions and messages effectively.

Severe Alienation:

- Continue to show presence through small gestures, cards, emails, or photos, regardless of response.
- Avoid expressing anger or despair directly to your child. They are caught in a system of coercion.
- Work through legal and therapeutic systems, while maintaining hope over time.

In all cases, never force conversations about the alienation itself. Focus on emotional availability and the child's internal world, not the alienating dynamics.

Recognising and Responding Strategically to Alienating Behaviours

You are not powerless, but acting wisely matters more than acting immediately.

- Document everything: Keep clear, chronological records of missed contact, hostile messages, or disparagement.
- Know when to escalate: Legal intervention is sometimes necessary, but timing and preparation are key.
- Avoid emotional traps: Alienating parents may bait you into looking unstable or aggressive. Always pause before responding.
- Control the narrative: Present a consistent, non-reactive presence, both in your child's eyes and in front of professionals.

Prioritising Parenting Time and Positive Contact

Even if conflict continues, never underestimate the healing power of positive time together.

- *Maximise opportunities* for shared routines, rituals, and joint activities, even short ones.
- *Use contact wisely*: Avoid interrogating your child about the other parent; focus on your connection.
- *Remain the adult*: Show resilience, flexibility, and warmth, even when you're hurting.

EMOTIONAL SURVIVAL: BUILDING RESILIENCE THROUGH THE JOURNEY

Parental alienation takes a profound emotional toll on targeted parents. It disrupts not only the relationship with one's child but also one's sense of identity, stability, and hope. Navigating this experience requires not just legal and strategic clarity, but emotional endurance. This section outlines core principles for maintaining emotional wellbeing, fostering resilience, and finding meaning and strength through adversity.

Acknowledging and Processing Emotion

- Validate your experience: The pain of being rejected by your child, especially unjustly, is real and deserving of attention.
- Permit grief: PA represents an ambiguous loss. Unlike bereavement, the child is alive and yet emotionally inaccessible. This can create cycles of hope, despair, anger, and guilt.
- Accept fluctuation: Emotional states may shift unpredictably; hope one week, despair the next. Recognising this as part of the process can reduce self-blame.

Developing and Maintaining Support Networks

- Prioritise connection: Isolation can deepen despair. Maintain regular contact with trusted friends, family, or support groups.
- Seek peer support: Connect with others who have experienced PA. The validation, advice, and solidarity can be transformative.
- Be discerning: Not everyone will understand PA. Engage with those who support your emotional safety, not those who dismiss or minimise your experience.

Coping Strategies and Self-Care Practices

- Mind–body care: Regular sleep, nutrition, and physical activity are foundational, not optional, for emotional resilience.
- Mindfulness and reflection: Practices like meditation, journalling, or gratitude lists can help ground you amid uncertainty.
- Constructive distraction: Pursuing hobbies or meaningful work can help reclaim a sense of self beyond the role of parent.

Engaging with Professional Help

- Therapists matter: Work with professionals familiar with PA and coercive control. General therapy may pathologise your reactions or misdiagnose the problem.

- Beware of unhelpful framing: If a professional tells you to "give the child space" without recognising the underlying manipulation, consider a second opinion.
- Use therapy strategically: As a space to process grief, rebuild self-worth, and develop long-term strategies for sustaining hope.

Rebuilding and Maintaining Relationships

- *Be patient and predictable*: Relationships may not improve quickly, but consistent, kind behaviour is your best foundation.
- *Create low-pressure moments*: If contact is possible, focus on everyday experiences – meals, walks, shared interests – rather than heavy conversations.
- *Model secure attachment*: Your child may be rejecting you, but your emotional steadiness can offer a blueprint for reconnection in the future.

Using Technology Wisely

- Stay present digitally: If physical contact is blocked, use email, texts, or recorded messages to show presence and care.
- Access resources: Online support groups, therapy platforms, and self-help tools can provide flexible and affordable support.
- Balance online and offline life: Avoid compulsive searches or over-engagement with conflict on social media. Set digital boundaries that protect your peace.

Supporting Children's Emotional Resilience

- Name the experience gently: Help your child understand they are not to blame for the alienation, using age-appropriate language.
- Encourage emotional expression: Teach your child to label and express emotions safely, whether in words, art, or movement.
- Connect through memories: When contact is limited, use stories, photos, or shared objects to maintain a sense of connection and continuity.
- Support their networks: Encourage relationships with safe, consistent adults, teachers, relatives, coaches, who can buffer against polarised narratives.
- Champion long-term healing: Even if reconnection is impossible now, nurture the conditions for future repair.

SUMMARY

Parental alienation presents not only legal and relational challenges but a sustained emotional ordeal for targeted parents. This chapter outlined key principles to support both practical navigation and emotional survival across the entire journey of PA. From co-parenting strategies and communication with resistant children to building a strong support network and managing the psychological impact of rejection, the emphasis is on agency, resilience, and connection. Emotional wellbeing is sustained through self-care, therapeutic support, peer validation, and patience. Though the path is often painful and protracted, targeted parents can retain their integrity, protect their hope, and lay the groundwork for eventual healing and reconnection.

21

GENERAL ADVICE FOR OTHER FAMILY MEMBERS, NEW PARTNERS, AND FRIENDS

Parental alienation reverberates across an entire network of relationships. Grandparents, extended family members, new partners, and close friends often find themselves affected by the dynamics of alienation, whether through being cut off from a child, witnessing the emotional toll on a loved one, or struggling to know how best to help. This chapter offers guidance for those on the periphery of an alienated family, clarifying how they can provide meaningful support, maintain hope, and avoid inadvertently reinforcing the alienation. By understanding the complex emotional landscape and adopting sensitive, informed strategies, these individuals can play a vital role in sustaining targeted parents and, when appropriate, helping to preserve the child's wider relational world.

SUPPORTING AS A GRANDPARENT: NAVIGATING THE COMPLEXITIES OF ALIENATION

Grandparents hold a unique and often emotionally charged position in families affected by parental alienation. Whether you are the grandparent of the alienated parent, watching your child suffer and losing contact with your grandchildren, or the grandparent of the alienating parent, potentially witnessing problematic behaviour or being drawn into conflict, your role

DOI: 10.4324/9781003630944-27

carries weight. Here's how you can navigate this difficult landscape with care, clarity, and compassion.

For Grandparents of the Alienated Parent

- Stay Visible and Loving: Even if you are cut off from your grandchildren, continue to express your love in age-appropriate, non-invasive ways, such as letters, cards, gifts, or messages that communicate stability and warmth without pressure. These may be rejected now, but they often matter deeply in the long run.
- Support Without Fueling Conflict: Avoid badmouthing the alienating parent or expressing anger in ways that could be weaponised against your child. Instead, focus on affirming your grandchild's right to love and be loved by both sides of their family.
- Be a Pillar for Your Adult Child: The pain of being alienated from one's child can be overwhelming. Offer your child non-judgmental support, encourage them to look after their mental health, and remind them that they are not alone in this experience.
- Document Carefully: Keep a calm, factual record of denied contact, changes in behaviour, or hostile interactions, should this information be helpful in legal or therapeutic contexts.
- Maintain Hope: Reunification is possible, even after years of estrangement. Stay steady, informed, and ready to reconnect when the opportunity arises.

For Grandparents of the Alienating Parent

- Examine Your Role: Reflect honestly on whether you may be consciously or unconsciously supporting alienating behaviours, such as siding openly with your adult child, vilifying the other parent, or restricting contact with the other side of the family.
- Prioritise the Grandchild's Needs: Remember that children benefit from safe, loving relationships with both parents and wider family. Enabling alienation, even out of loyalty to your own child, may contribute to long-term psychological harm for your grandchild.
- Encourage Healthy Boundaries: If your adult child is struggling with unresolved conflict or bitterness, gently encourage them to seek support. Alienation often stems from pain, but that does not excuse harmful behaviours.
- Be a Bridge, Not a Barrier: Where safe and appropriate, advocate for reconciliation and open dialogue. Sometimes, a neutral, trusted grandparent can model balanced thinking and help reduce polarisation within the family system.

Grandparents are often caught in the emotional crossfire of alienation, but they also hold great potential for healing and hope. Whether you're advocating quietly behind the scenes or waiting patiently for the door to reopen, your steadiness, compassion, and clarity can make a lasting difference.

SUPPORTING FROM THE SIDELINES: GUIDANCE FOR EXTENDED FAMILY MEMBERS

Extended family – aunts, uncles, cousins, and close family friends – often play important but overlooked roles in families impacted by parental alienation. You may be observing painful dynamics from a distance, unsure how to help without making things worse. Whether you are connected to the alienated parent or the alienating parent, your actions and attitudes can significantly influence the situation.

If You Are Connected to the Alienated Parent

- Affirm Their Pain Without Escalation: Listen empathetically and validate the alienated parent's grief and frustration, but avoid encouraging retaliatory behaviour or increasing hostility. Your calm presence can offer crucial grounding.
- Stay Present for the Child (If Possible): If you still have access to the alienated child, avoid withdrawing even if the relationship becomes strained or awkward. Continue to show warmth and support in neutral, non-threatening ways, such as brief messages, birthday cards, or gentle invitations.
- Avoid Negative Talk About the Other Parent: As tempting as it may be, criticising the alienating parent, especially around children, can reinforce the child's defences and deepen their sense of divided loyalty. Focus instead on your love for the child and your role as a constant, safe figure.
- Support Without Judgment: Alienated parents are often under intense emotional strain. Be patient, offer practical help, and remind them they are not to blame for their child's behaviour.

If You Are Connected to the Alienating Parent

- Reflect on Your Influence: Consider whether you may be contributing, directly or indirectly, to the child's rejection of the other parent, through sarcasm, taking sides, or reinforcing one-sided narratives.
- Encourage Accountability and Perspective: If it feels safe, try gently questioning assumptions or comments that dehumanise or vilify the other parent. Encourage your relative (the alienating parent) to prioritise the child's wellbeing over unresolved adult conflict.
- Be a Voice for Balance: You don't have to "choose sides" to be helpful. A calm, non-aligned approach can model to children and adults alike

that family relationships don't have to be defined by conflict or division.

- Protect the Child's Right to Love Both Parents: Extended family can play a powerful role in affirming that it is both safe and normal for a child to love both of their parents, regardless of adult disagreements.

Extended family members often feel powerless in the face of alienation, but your presence matters. Whether you're quietly offering support behind the scenes or holding space for future healing, your steadiness, kindness, and refusal to escalate conflict can offer children and parents a vital thread of connection and hope.

NAVIGATING WITH CARE: THE ROLE OF NEW PARTNERS IN ALIENATED FAMILIES

New partners often find themselves in emotionally complex and high-conflict environments when entering a family system affected by PA. Whether you are the partner of the alienated parent or the alienating parent, your position requires immense emotional intelligence, patience, and self-awareness. While the situation is not of your making, your influence, positive or negative, can be profound.

New Partners of Alienated Parents

Entering a relationship with someone whose child has been alienated from them presents unique emotional and relational challenges. You may witness their heartbreak, endure strained family interactions, and feel helpless in the face of injustice.
What You Can Do:

- Be a Steady Emotional Anchor: Offer emotional validation and support, not problem-solving. Understand that your partner is grieving a living loss, the rejection of their child, and that this grief is often cyclical and triggered by events like holidays, birthdays, or legal proceedings.
- Avoid Becoming the Spokesperson: However invested you are, it's crucial that you do not take on the role of advocate, defender, or challenger to the alienating parent or others involved. Your voice, if seen as combative or overbearing, can escalate conflict and be used as further ammunition to alienate the child.
- Don't Compete for Emotional Space: Understand that your partner's priority may often be their child, even when that child is currently rejecting them. Rather than seeing this as a threat, see it as a reflection of your partner's deep capacity for love, which likely extends to you as well.
- Respect the Child's Readiness: If there is ever an opportunity for reunification, tread lightly. Do not expect the child to immediately accept you

or treat you as a family member. Give space for the biological parent to re-establish the bond first, and only gradually, and respectfully, build your own connection.

- Take Care of Yourself: The emotional toll of supporting someone through PA can be high. Seek your own support network or counselling if needed. Protecting your wellbeing allows you to better support your partner long-term.

New Partners of Alienating Parents

In some cases, new partners of alienating parents may unintentionally, or intentionally, reinforce alienating behaviours. You may have entered the relationship hearing only one side of the story, and over time, find yourself drawn into patterns of rejection or vilification of the other parent.
What You Can Do:

- Approach with Curiosity and Caution: Be willing to consider that the narrative you've been told may be partial or distorted. Alienating parents often present themselves as victims and the other parent as dangerous or neglectful. Before forming firm judgments, ask: *What would this look like from the other side?*
- Refuse to Be Weaponised: If you are encouraged to speak badly about the other parent, block access, or interfere in communication between them and the child, this is a red flag. Participating in alienating behaviour, knowingly or not, can cause long-term harm to the child and may even lead to legal consequences.
- Focus on the Child's Needs, Not Loyalty: Children benefit from having access to both loving parents when it is safe to do so. Resist any pressure to win the child's loyalty or to take sides. Instead, model healthy relationships and balanced perspectives.
- Be Honest With Yourself: If you find that your partner's behaviour towards their co-parent seems controlling, manipulative, or obsessive, reflect honestly on what this might indicate. Sometimes, new partners become enmeshed in toxic dynamics that cause harm to the child and strain their own wellbeing.

Shared Challenges and Responsibilities

Regardless of which side you are on, there are shared responsibilities that come with being a new partner in an alienated family:

- Model Respectful Communication: Whether speaking with the child, your partner, or others involved, model calm, respectful, and emotionally intelligent behaviour. Children are always watching and learning.

- Protect Children from Conflict: Never involve children in adult disputes, speak negatively about the other parent, or pressure them to disclose information. This includes avoiding subtle undermining or sarcastic remarks that may influence the child's views.
- Be Patient and Long-Term Focused: Alienation is rarely resolved quickly. It may take years for healing and reconnection to occur, if at all. Focus on building a family environment that feels safe, stable, and loving, without conditions.
- Know When to Step Back: In moments of high conflict, it may be best to step back from the centre of family negotiations or communication. Letting biological parents lead, when appropriate, can defuse tension and give space for direct parent–child repair.

New partners are often the "invisible actors" in alienation dynamics, yet their role is critical. You have the power to either deepen division or support healing, sometimes simply by doing less, listening more, and choosing compassion over control. By staying grounded, open-minded, and child-centred, you can help cultivate an environment where, one day, relationships may begin to rebuild.

FRIENDS, NEIGHBOURS, AND COMMUNITY: SUPPORTING WITH COMPASSION AND CLARITY

Parental alienation often unfolds behind closed doors, but its impact ripples outward; into friendships, workplaces, schools, places of worship, and community spaces. Friends, neighbours, and community members can be powerful allies in either perpetuating or challenging alienation dynamics, often without realising the influence they hold. Understanding how to respond with compassion, neutrality, and informed curiosity is essential.

Avoid Taking Sides Too Quickly

When one parent presents themselves as the victim of an "absent," "dangerous," or "disinterested" co-parent, it can be tempting to take them at their word, especially if you trust them. But alienation often involves narratives that are skewed, exaggerated, or untrue.

- Stay curious. Ask questions. Reflect on what you haven't heard.
- Withhold judgment unless you have direct evidence of abuse or neglect.
- Recognise complexity: even seemingly one-sided stories often have multiple layers.

Consider the Child's Perspective

Children in alienation dynamics may outwardly reject one parent while inwardly feeling confused, conflicted, or coerced. Their apparent "loyalty" to one parent may be a survival strategy or the result of long-term manipulation.

- Don't reinforce rejection by speaking negatively about the other parent in front of the child.
- Support a child's right to love both parents, where it is safe to do so.
- Be a safe, neutral presence, offering space where the child does not feel pressured to take sides.

Support Without Enabling

If your friend or relative is the alienating parent, it is still possible to be supportive while gently holding a mirror to their behaviour. Alienation thrives when the surrounding community validates its justifications or ignores red flags.

- Avoid amplifying grievances against the other parent, especially in front of the child.
- Encourage reflection: "Have you thought about how [the child] might feel not seeing their other parent?"
- Signpost to support rather than trying to solve the situation yourself.

If your friend or relative is the alienated parent, your role can be one of validation, encouragement, and constancy.

- Believe them: Alienation often goes unrecognised, and alienated parents may feel invisible or disbelieved.
- Be a witness to their efforts and pain, even when there's no immediate resolution.
- Offer practical help, whether it's a listening ear, help with legal paperwork, or time to rest.

Maintain Connection with the Child (When Appropriate)

If you are close to the child and have a long-standing relationship, maintaining contact can help preserve a sense of stability and serve as a bridge in future reconnection efforts.

- Be subtle and respectful: Don't confront the child or try to "correct" their views.
- Model balanced thinking by speaking positively or neutrally about both parents.
- Stay present in the child's life if possible, send birthday messages, show up at events, and remind them of your unconditional regard.

Use Your Influence Wisely

Friends and community members often have unique access to moments of reflection, especially when tensions are high.

- Challenge harmful assumptions about parenting roles, custody norms, or gendered stereotypes.
- Share resources: books, articles, or support groups may open up new understanding.
- Encourage professional input: Suggest involving a neutral mediator, therapist, or parenting expert when conversations become cyclical or combative.

In alienation scenarios, silence and neutrality can sometimes feel safest; however, thoughtful and informed engagement can make a real difference. By remaining compassionate yet grounded, friends and community members can support healthy relationships, reduce isolation, and serve as quiet counterweights to the polarisation that parental alienation creates. Your presence may not end the alienation, but it can help prevent further harm, and keep the door open to healing.

SUMMARY

This chapter explored the often-overlooked role of extended family, new partners, friends, and community members in cases of parental alienation. These individuals can significantly influence the family dynamic, either by reinforcing alienation or by helping to bridge the divide. Through tailored guidance, the chapter outlined how grandparents, aunts and uncles, step-parents, and friends can support both the alienated parent and the child in ways that are empathetic, non-judgmental, and child-centred. Emphasising the need for balanced thinking, respectful involvement, and informed support, the chapter underscored how meaningful social relationships outside the immediate parental conflict can contribute to resilience, healing, and the eventual restoration of family bonds.

22

ADVICE FOR CHILDREN; WRITTEN FOR THEM

Throughout this book, there have been little pieces of advice for children and young people like you; things to think about when you're feeling stuck, sad, angry, or confused about what's happening in your family. This chapter brings all of that together in one place. It's written just for you. You might be someone who's feeling caught in the middle, unsure who to trust, or like you're being asked to choose sides. Or maybe you're feeling distant from one of your parents and not quite sure why. Whatever you're feeling, you're not alone. This chapter will give you ideas to help you understand what's happening, look after yourself, and find your own way through. You don't need to have all the answers, but you do deserve support, kindness, and space to figure things out.

WHAT YOU CAN DO, WHAT YOU CAN FEEL, AND HOW YOU CAN FIND SUPPORT

When your parents separate, or when things get tense between them, it can feel scary, confusing, or lonely. If you're also going through something like parental alienation, where one parent is trying to stop or limit your relationship with the other parent, it can feel even more painful. This chapter brings together all the advice you've seen elsewhere and adds more, so you have a toolkit for understanding, coping, and getting support. You're not to blame

DOI: 10.4324/9781003630944-28

for what's happening, and there *are* things you can do and people you can lean on. Below are ideas and suggestions you can use, mix and match, or try when you feel ready.

It's Okay to Feel Whatever You're Feeling

- Your feelings – anger, sadness, confusion, guilt, and fear – are real, and they matter.
- You don't need to pretend to be "strong" all the time. Let yourself cry, yell, journal, draw, or talk it out.
- Some days you'll feel okay, some days you won't. That's normal. Feelings go up and down.

You Are Not Responsible

- You are *not* the reason your parents are separated or fighting.
- You do *not* have to choose one parent over the other. You deserve relationships with both, provided it's safe.
- You don't have to fix the problems or carry the emotional burden. That's for adults and professionals.

Talk with Someone You Trust

- Find someone you can share your feelings with – a friend, aunt, uncle, grandparent, teacher, counsellor, or coach.
- Choose someone who listens, doesn't judge you, and helps you feel safer, not more worried.
- You don't have to talk about everything all at once. You can say: "I'm having a hard time," and let them help you decide where to start.

Use Words That Help, Not Hurt

- When you talk, try using *I-statements*: "I feel sad when . . . ," "I'm worried that . . . ," "I wish . . ."
- If something someone said upsets you, you can say, "That word hurts me," or "Can we talk differently?"
- You don't have to be polite to hurtful words; if someone says something mean about one of your parents, you can say, "I'd prefer not to talk that way."

Keep Your Own Voice in the Story

- When people talk about your family, you don't always have to repeat what they say. You can say your own truth.

- If someone pressures you to take sides, you can say, "I need time to think about that," or "I'm not comfortable choosing between them."
- It's okay to change your mind as you grow and get more information.

Stay Connected Where You Can

- If you can, safely keep contact with both parents (or as much as the situation allows). It may help keep doors open for the future.
- Use letters, texts, pictures – ways to remind your parents you care, even if they can't always respond.
- Use in-person time wisely: do things you enjoy together, such as walks, shared meals, quiet time, or games, without pressure or needing to "fix" the relationship.

Build Your Own Support System

- Befriend people outside the conflict: friends, coaches, team members, neighbours.
- Join clubs, teams, or groups you like: sports, art, music, drama, whatever interests you. They can be a refuge.
- If there's a school counsellor, social worker, or mental health professional, reach out. You don't have to go through it alone.

Take Care of Yourself (Mind, Body, Spirit)

- Sleep, good food, and exercise all help when your brain is under stress.
- Do things you love: music, drawing, reading, nature, writing, and playing with a pet.
- Try relaxing activities: breathing, mindfulness, short walks, and stretching to calm your mind when things feel overwhelming.

Ask Questions When You're Unsure

- If adults make decisions about your life (school, extra activities, where you live), ask, "Why is this happening?" or "How does it help me?"
- If things feel unfair to you, or someone's being hurtful, ask for help to understand or to speak up. You deserve respect.
- You can ask for a meeting with a counsellor, therapist, or mediator to help you understand decisions and feel heard.

Hold On to Hope, But Be Realistic

- Healing and reconnection often takes time. It may not happen quickly, and sometimes there are setbacks. But that doesn't mean it's impossible.

- Many people who've been through alienation later look back and see how certain actions, small kindnesses, consistent presence, and emotional steadiness mattered.
- Even if things don't fully go "back to normal," your life can still stay meaningful, you can build new relationships, and you can grow stronger from what you experience.

Safety First

- If at any time you are in danger, feel unsafe, or someone is threatening you or another parent, tell a trusted adult immediately – teacher, school counsellor, social worker, police.
- If someone pressures you to do or say things you don't want to, that's not okay. You have a right to your own voice and boundaries.

You're not invisible. Your feelings, your voice, and your future matter. The love you've had, the dreams you still carry, the resilience you're building – they're real and meaningful. Even when it's hard to see, you have worth and you deserve to be cared for, to grow, and to heal. This path may be rocky, but you don't have to walk it alone.

CONCLUSION

Parental alienation is not a myth, a mere parenting conflict, or a superficial custody dispute. It is a form of emotional abuse grounded in coercive relational dynamics. As this book has sought to demonstrate, the scientific evidence supports PA's validity, and it clearly inflicts real psychological, developmental, and relational harm on children and parents alike. Recognising PA as abuse is thus not a rhetorical flourish; it is a necessary first step towards ensuring victims are not dismissed or disbelieved and that interventions are taken seriously.

The urgency of addressing PA cannot be overstated. The effects reverberate far beyond the immediate trauma: children exposed to sustained alienation often suffer identity disruption, emotional dysregulation, attachment fragmentation, and long-term relational difficulties. For parents, the pain is often one of ambiguous loss, complex grief, and abuse to the core of their parental identity. If left unchecked, PA can span generations, undermining trust, family continuity, and psychological flourishing. To prevent and repair these harms, systemic and intentional responses are essential.

No single actor can carry this burden alone. Schools, health services, legal and court systems, social work and child welfare agencies, media, communities, and cultural institutions all have roles to play. Schools must become safe detection and support hubs; courts must embed PA expertise and enforceable remedies; social workers must adopt curiosity and refusal to

DOI: 10.4324/9781003630944-29

collude; media must shift from sensationalism to sensitive portrayal; communities must reaffirm children's rights to both parents. Only when every level of the ecosystem is engaged can we transform the conditions that allow PA to flourish.

That transformation demands systemic change. Laws should explicitly recognise PA within abuse or coercive control frameworks. Legal mechanisms must be strengthened so that court orders are meaningful and enforceable. Professional training, across psychology, social work, education, and law, must include PA as a core competency. Public policies should incentivise early intervention, shared parenting models, and cross-system collaboration. Awareness campaigns, media guidelines, and cultural education must challenge the norms that excuse exclusion or reward parental gatekeeping. It is not enough to respond; we must reshape the ecosystem so that PA becomes less likely, less tolerated, and more swiftly addressed.

Yet, even against these formidable challenges, there is real hope. *To alienated parents,* I offer this: your persistence, dignity, and love are not in vain. Even in seasons of silence, your presence matters. Your self-care, clear documentation, and readiness to repair plant seeds of possibility. *To alienated children,* I wish you courage: your voice, autonomy, and inner truth are yours to reclaim. When safe, relationships can be rebuilt, and narratives reframed. Many who were once alienated later remember and resonate with parental gestures of consistency and love; those gestures matter.

As we look ahead, let us commit together:

- to validate PA as a serious form of psychological harm;
- to demand institutional accountability and systemic change;
- to build supportive infrastructures in every community;
- and to nurture hope, healing, and reconnection whenever possible.

May this work contribute to a future in which no child is silenced, no parent is erased, and families, even imperfect ones, can heal, grow, and remain generative across time.

APPENDICES

Appendix A – Other Books on PA

Baker, A. J. (2010). *Adult children of parental alienation syndrome: Breaking the ties that bind.* WW Norton & Company.

Baker, A. J., & Fine, P. R. (2017). *Surviving parental alienation: A journey of hope and healing.* Rowman & Littlefield Publishers.

Graham, S. (2023). *Attachment-led theory and practice in parental alienation.* Independently Published.

Haines, J., Matthewson, M., & Turnbull, M. (2019). *Understanding and managing parental alienation: A guide to assessment and intervention.* Routledge.

Hine, B. A. (2023). *Parental alienation: A contemporary guide for parents, practitioners, and policymakers.* Independently Published.

Kig, S., & Shama, F. (2022). *A practical guide to parental alienation in private and public law children cases.* Law Brief Publishing.

Kneier, G. (2021). *Parental alienation: A child-psychology approach: It is a denial of attachment.* Amazon.

Laquidara, D. (2023). *YOU-KNOW-WHO: An alienated daughter's memoir.* Independently Published.

Lorandos, D., & Bernet, W. (Eds.). (2020). *Parental alienation: Science and law.* Charles C Thomas Publisher, Ltd.

Lorandos, D., Bernet, W., & Sauber, S. R. (2013). *Parental alienation: The handbook for mental health and legal professionals* (Vol. 1116). Charles C Thomas Publisher, Ltd.

McCarten, D. (2022). *Parental alienation: An evidence-based approach.* Routledge.

Shubert, D. R. (2023). *Parental alienation unmasked: Understanding, coping, and moving forward as a family.* Independently Published.

Warshak, R. A. (2001). *Divorce poison: Protecting the parent-child bond from a vindictive ex* (p. 320). ReganBooks.

Woodall, K., & Woodall, N. (2017). *Understanding parental alienation: Learning to cope, helping to heal.* Charles C Thomas Publisher, Ltd.

Appendix B – Sources of Additional Support

Below is a list of support groups and organisations that provide support to alienated parents as well as further resources to educate on this topic:

1. Families Need Fathers (FNF) – A charity that helps parents maintain a meaningful relationship with their children following a separation or divorce. They provide information, support, and guidance to parents dealing with parental alienation.
   Website: https://fnf.org.uk/
2. The Parental Alienation Study Group (PASG) – An international, non-profit organization dedicated to raising awareness, providing education, and promoting research on parental alienation. They have members in the UK who can provide support and resources to alienated parents.
   Website: https://pasg.info/
3. Parental Alienation UK – Has a resources section on their website, which includes online resources and organizations related to parental alienation. They invite users to email them with additional resources they find helpful, aiming to provide comprehensive support.
   Website: https://parentalalienationuk.info/
3. Parental Alienation Europe (PAE) – A network of professionals and volunteers working together to raise awareness, educate, and provide support to those affected by parental alienation across Europe, including the UK.
   Website: https://www.parental-alienation-europe.com/
4. MatchMothers – A UK-based charity that offers support to non-resident mothers experiencing difficulties in maintaining contact with their

children following separation or divorce. They provide advice, support, and a listening ear to mothers facing parental alienation.
Website: https://www.matchmothers.org/

5. National Association of Alienated Parents (NAAP) – A UK-based organization that provides support, advice, and advocacy for parents experiencing parental alienation. They offer resources, workshops, and conferences to help parents navigate the challenges of parental alienation.
Website: https://alienatedparents.org.uk/
6. Voice of the Child – A UK-based organization that offers information, resources, and support to parents and professionals dealing with high-conflict divorce, separation, and parental alienation.
Website: https://voiceofthechild.org.uk/
7. Child Access and Prevention of Parental Alienation (CAPPA) – A UK-based organization that provides information, support, and resources for parents dealing with parental alienation and child access issues.
Website: https://www.cappa.co.uk/
8. Cafcass (Children and Family Court Advisory and Support Service) provides information on their position regarding parental alienation, offering insight into how the organization approaches cases involving this issue.
Website: https://www.cafcass.gov.uk/
9. Parental Alienation Awareness Organization (PAAO): An international organization aiming to raise awareness about Parental Alienation. They provide resources, support, and organize an annual Parental Alienation Awareness Day.
Website: https://www.paawareness.org/
10. Shared Parenting Council of Australia: A non-profit organization aiming to ensure children have the right to love and be loved by both parents, and to ensure children have the opportunity for both parents to be involved in their lives.
Website: http://www.spca.org.au/
11. Erasing Family: A non-profit aiming to reunite children with their erased parents by promoting family bond obstruction reform. They offer resources and support for erased family members.
Website: https://erasingfamily.org/
12. Simply Parent: A non-profit organization aiming to support and empower parents and their allies who face parental alienation, false allegations, and other forms of family bond obstruction.
Website: https://simplyparent.org/
13. Family Access – Fighting for Children's Rights: An organization providing support and resources for families dealing with issues such as divorce, custody, visitation, and parental alienation.
Website: http://www.familyaccessfightingforchildrensrights.com/

The UK also offers several legal resources for alienated parents seeking help, information, or representation. Here are some of them:

1. Resolution: This is a community of family justice professionals who are committed to a constructive, non-confrontational approach to family law issues. Their website provides a directory of solicitors and other professionals who can provide legal advice or representation in cases of parental alienation.
   Website: http://www.resolution.org.uk/
2. Citizens Advice: They offer free, confidential, and impartial advice on a range of legal issues, including family law and child custody disputes. They can also provide guidance on finding a solicitor.
   Website: https://www.citizensadvice.org.uk/
3. Family Law Bar Association: They represent barristers who specialise in family law. They can provide resources on understanding family law and can help you find a barrister who specialises in parental alienation cases.
   Website: https://www.flba.co.uk/
4. The Law Society: They offer a "Find a Solicitor" service, which can be used to find legal professionals specialising in family law and parental alienation cases.
   Website: https://solicitors.lawsociety.org.uk/
5. Child Law Advice: Run by Coram Children's Legal Centre, it provides specialist advice and information on child, family and education law to parents, carers, and young people in England.
   Website: https://childlawadvice.org.uk/
6. Family Law Panel: A directory of family law solicitors who follow a code of practice that promotes a constructive and ethical approach to family law matters, including parental alienation.
   Website: https://thefamilylawpanel.org/
   Always remember to seek professional advice when dealing with legal matters. It is important to find a solicitor who is familiar with parental alienation and can help navigate the complexities of family law.
   Here are additional resources for various countries:
   United States:
7. American Bar Association: Provides a comprehensive directory of family law attorneys across the United States.
   Website: https://www.americanbar.org/
8. Legal Services Corporation: Offers legal aid to individuals with low-income.
   Website: https://www.lsc.gov/
9. National Association of Counsel for Children: Specializes in law related to children.
   Website: https://www.nacchildlaw.org/
   Australia:

10. Legal Aid NSW: Provides free or low-cost legal aid services in New South Wales.
    Website: https://www.legalaid.nsw.gov.au/
11. Family Law Section of the Law Council of Australia: Represents family law practitioners and offers resources on family law matters.
    Website: https://www.familylawsection.org.au/
    Canada:
12. Legal Aid Ontario: Provides access to legal aid services for low-income individuals.
    Website: https://www.legalaid.on.ca/
13. Canadian Bar Association: Offers a directory to find lawyers who specialize in various areas of law, including family law.
    Website: https://www.cba.org/
    South Africa:
14. Legal Aid South Africa: Provides professional legal advice and representation to those who can't afford it.
    Website: https://legal-aid.co.za/
15. Law Society of South Africa: Offers a directory to find lawyers and other legal resources.
    Website: https://www.lssa.org.za/
    India:
16. Legal Services Authorities Act 1987: Provides free legal services to weaker sections of society. Reach out to the local District Legal Services Authority.
17. National Legal Services Authority: Responsible for providing free legal aid in civil and criminal matters for the poor and marginalised people who can't afford the services of a lawyer.
    Website: https://nalsa.gov.in/

Please note that legal systems can differ greatly by country, and parental alienation may not be recognised or treated the same way everywhere. Always ensure to find a legal professional who is knowledgeable about parental alienation in your specific jurisdiction.

Appendix C – Common PA FAQs

1. **What is parental alienation (PA)?**
   Parental alienation occurs when a child unjustifiably rejects or resists a relationship with one parent (the targeted parent), typically due to manipulation, pressure, or influence by the other parent (the alienating parent). This rejection is not explained by abuse, neglect, or deficient parenting, but arises from a sustained pattern of alienating behaviours.
2. **What are the signs and behaviours associated with PA?**
   Warning signs may include a child:
   - expressing unjustified hostility, fear, or rejection towards one parent,
   - echoing the alienating parent's negative views,
   - refusing contact without clear cause,
   - showing a lack of ambivalence (seeing one parent as all "good" and the other as all "bad"), or
   - withdrawing affection if they maintain contact with the targeted parent.

   Alienating behaviours can include denigrating the other parent, limiting or interfering with contact, withholding information, creating fear or guilt around loving the targeted parent, and enlisting others to reinforce the rejection.
3. **How is PA viewed legally in the UK and internationally?**
   UK family courts recognise that alienation can harm children, and judges increasingly consider it in custody disputes. However, PA is not defined in statute. Internationally, recognition varies: some jurisdictions explicitly acknowledge PA as abuse, while others are more cautious.

4. **How can PA be evidenced in court?**
Demonstrating PA is complex. Courts often require professional assessments by psychologists or social workers. Parents can assist by documenting incidents, maintaining consistent efforts to engage with the child, and working with legal professionals familiar with PA.
5. **What should I do if I suspect alienation?**
Seek early advice from legal and mental health professionals who understand PA. Avoid retaliating or criticising the other parent in front of your child. Focus on maintaining calm, consistent, loving contact where possible.
6. **Can PA be reversed?**
Yes, although it is challenging. Recovery often requires therapeutic intervention, rebuilding trust over time, and sometimes legal action to safeguard the parent–child relationship. Outcomes vary depending on severity, the child's age, and the responsiveness of the system.
7. **How does PA affect children, both now and later in life?**
Children may experience anxiety, depression, low self-esteem, identity confusion, and difficulties with trust. Many feel guilt or regret as they mature and recognise the manipulation. These patterns can affect adult relationships, increasing vulnerability to conflict and unhealthy dynamics.
8. **Is PA considered a form of abuse?**
Many professionals regard severe PA as a form of emotional abuse, because it distorts a child's reality, damages attachment bonds, and inflicts long-term psychological harm.
9. **Does PA only happen after divorce or separation?**
No. Although most common in separated families, alienation can also occur in intact families where one parent fosters hostility or fear towards the other.
10. **What professional or community support is available?**
Support may come from family therapists, child psychologists, solicitors, specialist organisations, and peer support groups. A multidisciplinary approach – legal, psychological, and emotional – usually works best. (See Appendix B for resources.)
11. **How can I communicate with my child during alienation?**
Always maintain a stance of unconditional love. Avoid criticising the other parent to the child. Stay calm and patient, offering reassurance that the child is loved and safe with you, even if responses are minimal or negative.
12. **How can I protect or rebuild my relationship with my child?**
Consistency is vital. Continue age-appropriate efforts at contact (direct or indirect, as legally permitted), record attempts, and seek guidance from professionals. Encourage open communication and avoid placing blame on the child.

13. **How long does alienation last, and can children recover fully?**
There is no fixed timeline. Recovery depends on the degree of alienation, the effectiveness of interventions, and the support available. Many children can and do heal, but the process may take years.
14. **Can alienating parents change?**
Yes, but only with recognition of the harm caused and usually with professional or legal intervention. Change is often difficult if the alienating parent denies the problem.
15. **What if the court does not recognise my concerns about PA?**
Engage an experienced solicitor, consider expert psychological input, and persist with gathering and presenting evidence. Even if progress is slow, sustained advocacy can make a difference.
16. **What if I face accusations of abuse (true or false)?**
Allegations of abuse, whether founded or unfounded, complicate alienation cases. Legal advice is critical. If accusations are false, gather evidence and comply with investigations. If they are true, participation in interventions or programmes may be required before contact can resume.
17. **What if I am subject to restricted or no-contact orders?**
Comply fully with any court order to avoid worsening the situation. For indirect contact, continue sending loving messages. For no-contact, work with your solicitor to seek reassessment when possible. Demonstrating patience, compliance, and ongoing commitment can strengthen your position.
18. **How is PA different from estrangement or loyalty conflicts?**
    - *Alienation* arises from one parent's manipulation leading to unjustified rejection.
    - *Estrangement* reflects a child's justified rejection due to the targeted parent's behaviour (e.g., abuse, neglect).
    - *Loyalty conflicts* occur when a child feels torn between parents without necessarily rejecting either one.
19. **Does PA have degrees of severity?**
Yes, it is commonly understood as mild, moderate, or severe. Interventions differ according to intensity, with severe cases often requiring more robust legal or therapeutic measures.
20. **Is PAS the same as PA?**
Parental Alienation Syndrome (PAS), introduced in the 1980s, described a cluster of child behaviours linked to alienation. It has been widely criticised for weak evidence and is not included in the DSM–5. Today, most professionals focus on PA as a behavioural and relational problem, rather than a psychiatric syndrome.
21. **Do children repeat alienating behaviours as adults?**
Some do. Growing up in an environment where manipulation and rejection are normalised can increase the risk of repeating these patterns in their own relationships.

22. **Can mediation help?**
Mediation may help in mild or early cases, provided the mediator understands PA. In entrenched or severe cases, mediation alone is unlikely to resolve the problem and could even reinforce harmful dynamics.
23. **Who else is affected by PA?**
Alienation can fracture a child's relationships not only with the targeted parent, but also with grandparents, siblings, and the wider family. Schools may also be drawn in, sometimes unknowingly reinforcing alienation through exclusion of the targeted parent.
24. **What role can schools and professionals play?**
Schools and professionals can provide valuable observations, ensure both parents are informed about a child's progress (where appropriate), and avoid being drawn into one-sided narratives. Training in recognising PA can improve responses.
25. **Are there support groups or communities for alienated families?**
Yes. Many national and local organisations offer peer groups, online forums, and helplines for alienated parents and extended families. These provide emotional support, advocacy, and practical advice.
26. **Can PA be prevented?**
Prevention is possible by promoting cooperative co-parenting, encouraging healthy attachment to both parents, addressing early signs of alienating behaviour, and ensuring legal and professional systems intervene promptly when concerns arise.

Appendix D – 15 Common Myths About Parental Alienation

Myth 1: Parental alienation is not real

Some still claim parental alienation (PA) is not a legitimate phenomenon. In reality, a large body of research and clinical evidence demonstrates that PA exists and can have profound effects on children and families.

Myth 2: Parental alienation is rare or unusual

PA is not uncommon. Prevalence varies, but it has been documented in many countries, across socio-economic groups, and in both high- and low-conflict families.

Myth 3: Only high-conflict divorces cause PA

Although more visible in separation and divorce, PA can also occur in intact families. The critical factor is the behaviour of an alienating parent, not the family structure.

Myth 4: Only mothers (or only fathers) alienate

Both mothers and fathers can engage in alienating behaviours. PA is not gender-specific.

Myth 5: Alienation is the child's fault

Children are never to blame. Their rejection of one parent reflects psychological manipulation and pressure they are unable to resist.

Myth 6: Only bad or neglectful parents are alienated

Even caring, competent parents may be alienated. Alienation reflects the alienating parent's actions and motives, not the targeted parent's quality of care.

Myth 7: If a child rejects a parent, it must mean the parent did something wrong

While children may reject parents for legitimate reasons (e.g., abuse or neglect), PA is different. In alienation, the rejection is unjustified and disproportionate.

Myth 8: Parental alienation is harmless or short-lived

PA is emotionally damaging and often considered a form of psychological abuse. Its effects can last well into adulthood, shaping self-esteem, trust, and relationships.

Myth 9: PA is easy to spot and simple to prove

Alienation can be subtle and disguised as normal child behaviour. It usually requires professional assessment to distinguish from estrangement or loyalty conflicts.

Myth 10: Children will simply "grow out of it"

Without intervention, the consequences of alienation can persist long-term. Many alienated children carry the effects into adult relationships and identity.

Myth 11: Parental alienation can be resolved quickly or without help

Rebuilding relationships after alienation takes time, patience, and usually professional or legal intervention. It is not solved by goodwill alone.

Myth 12: Accusations of parental alienation are always genuine

Not all claims are valid. Sometimes false allegations are raised to gain advantage in custody disputes. Careful, evidence-based assessment is essential.

Myth 13: Courts always recognise and respond effectively to PA

Legal systems vary widely. Some judges lack training in PA, and inconsistent responses can worsen the problem. Determining PA in court often requires expert testimony and can be lengthy.

Myth 14: PA only involves direct badmouthing of a parent

Alienation takes many forms, including limiting contact, undermining authority, creating fear or guilt, or manipulating extended family and professionals against the targeted parent.

Myth 15: Parental alienation is confined to certain cultures or societies

PA has been identified worldwide, in diverse cultural, economic, and social contexts. While cultural factors shape how it appears and is addressed, no group is immune.

Index

For Product Safety Concerns and Information please contact our
EU representative GPSR@taylorandfrancis.com Taylor & Francis
Verlag GmbH, Kaufingerstraße 24, 80331 München, Germany